D0106048

"*To reach from within the place of great suffering—and not to a means of escape, but to Jesus—is rare. The multi-storied pages of this book tell of that kind of woman, one with a deep reach for the Jesus who moves through every single tear. Jenna's story radiates Jesus, and her husband's outpouring, while dealing with his great loss, is a moving testimony of beauty.*"

SARA HAGERTY, author of *Every Bitter Thing is Sweet* and *Unseen: The Gift of Being Hidden in a World that Loves to be Noticed*

"*Worth the Suffering tells the story of a woman who wasn't playing for just her 30 years here on Earth, she was playing for eternity and that was evident in the intentionality of the life she lived. Jenna's prayers and journal entries captured in this book will strengthen your faith, wherever you are in that journey and offer you the same hope that Jenna's life was rooted in.*"

BRIAN TOME, founding and Senior Pastor of Crossroads Church, author of *Welcome to the Revolution*, *Five Marks of a Man* and *Free Book*

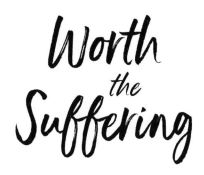

Worth
*the*
Suffering

# Worth the Suffering

## LOVING & LEAVING THIS LIFE

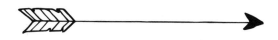

*jenna henderson*

*Worth the Suffering: Loving & Leaving This Life*

Copyright © 2017 by Jenna Henderson

All rights reserved. Unless designated, no part of this book may be reproduced in any form, except for brief quotations in reviews, without the written permission of the Publisher.

Unless otherwise indicated, all Scriptures quotations are from the Holy Bible, English Standard Version, copyright © 2001 by Crossway Bibles, a publishing ministry of Good News Publishers. Used by permission. All rights reserved.

Scripture quotations marked *(NIV)* are taken from the *HOLY BIBLE, NEW INTERNATIONAL VERSION®, NIV®*, Copyright © 1973, 1978, 1984, 2011 by Biblica, Inc.® Used by permission of Zondervan. All rights reserved worldwide.

Scripture quotations marked (NLT) are taken from the Holy Bible, New Living Translation, copyright © 1996, 2004, 2007, 2013, 2015 by Tyndale House Foundation. Used by permission of Tyndale House Publishers, Inc., Carol Stream, Illinois 60188. All rights reserved.

Published by Distressed Roots LLC
Batesville, Indiana
www.distressedroots.com

Production assistance by Winters Publishing
Greensburg, Indiana
www.winterspublishing.com

Library of Congress Control Number: 2017919014

ISBN: 978-0-692-98344-7

*Cover art by Leah Henderson*
*Hand-drawn arrows and waves by Marissa Cupp*
*Logo design by Dan Royer Designs*

Printed in the United States of America

*In loving memory of my wife*

*Jenna Henderson*

# Contents

# Exhale

# Crashing Waves

# Foreword

Life is different now. Every step forward feels like it is taking me further and further away from the life I always envisioned. A life filled with years of joyful, adventurous moments with my wife as we learned what it meant to live life together. A life where we fulfilled our dreams of starting a family and where we fully lived out the rest of our days together.

Never did I imagine that only 3 years into my marriage with my wife, Jenna, we would receive devastating, life-altering news. It started with an all-too-familiar abdominal pain and confirmed with elevated lab results. After 13 years of being in remission, Jenna's ovarian cancer had returned. This would be the start of her third (and eventually, fourth) bout with cancer at the young age of 28.

How are you supposed to respond when you hear the doctor utter these words? How do you have faith when God seems so absent from a situation? What do you do when your entire future gets erased by one tragic event?

Over the next year and a half, I had the heartrending blessing to watch Jenna fully answer these questions as she gracefully fought this horrendous disease. In October of 2016, I sat next to my wife and held her hand as she took her last breath and left this unforgiving world broken; only to be received into her Father's arms wholly healed and restored.

I call this a blessing because even in the midst of my worst nightmare, I received so many priceless gifts that can only be uncovered through suffering. When reality sets in that life isn't promised, it greatly changes things. Jenna and I were able to share more sweet, tender moments in that year and a half than many married couples do in a lifetime. I was able to fully grasp and experience real, authentic love—not what the world tries to define love as. I discovered what sacrificially serving the one you love will do to your heart. To me, these (and many more unmentioned) are those gifts.

It is an honor to share with you a gift she left to us all. Through her suffering, Jenna wrote many blogs and prayers about what it is like to go through something so tragic, yet convey so much joy and hope because of her faith in Jesus.

This book takes us through a timeline of Jenna's journey while integrating stories from her friends throughout her life. As you read, you will notice arrows, leaves, and waves. The arrows signify her writings, the leaves her prayers, and the waves (with a gray box in the background), a story shared by a friend.

Many of Jenna's writings, as well as those stories you will read from friends, mention the ministry of Young Life. This was central to who she was and how she lived, so I find it important to share with you all a little more about it.

———

At its core, Young Life's mission is to introduce adolescents to Jesus Christ and help them grow in their faith. Yet somehow, this doesn't fully capture the depth and beauty of this ministry.

It starts with adults who are concerned enough about kids to go to them, on their turf and in their culture, building bridges of authentic friendship. These relationships don't happen overnight—they take time, patience, trust, and consistency.

Young Life leaders log many hours with kids—where they are, as they are. They listen to the students' stories and genuinely care about their joys, triumphs, heartaches, and setbacks. They share the good news about who Jesus is in a language they can understand, and love them regardless of their response to it. These leaders are willing to enter the world of teenagers who are hurting, broken, written-off, vulgar and reckless, lost and forgotten, enslaved by substances, ignored or abandoned, in order to walk with them and love them for who they are.[1]

———

Life is much simpler now. Things that are truly important in this life are far easier to notice and far easier to live out. Jenna's life, and her death, reflect what it looks like to cling to Jesus even when it feels like God is nowhere to be found. Her life, *especially in that last year and a half*, radiated the love, joy, peace, patience, kindness, goodness, faithfulness, gentleness, and self-control promised in Galatians 5:22.[2]

You may feel like God has abandoned you in your suffering (or even your day-to-day overwhelmed and busy life). You may feel alone, betrayed, confused, and uncertain. But after living through this suffering with Jenna, I am certain of this now more so than ever—there is nothing on this Earth more important, more comforting, or more life-giving, than knowing and fully trusting Jesus.

I mean the real Jesus, maybe not the unattractive one you learned about in Sunday school, but the One who promises you a full, adventure-filled life. The One who promises to never leave or forsake you. The One who reminds us our life is short, yet there is so much more waiting for you on the other side. The One who promises that He will wipe every tear from your eyes, defeat death, and joyfully celebrate his sons and daughters when they return home.

*– Scott*

## FIRST SEASON

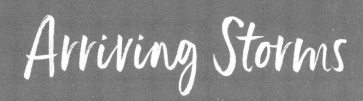

# Arriving Storms

# Only the beginning

What is it like to stare down death, but not be scared? If I'm completely honest, I feared death prior to Jenna's passing. Death encompassed this great unknown, and the fear that the life I knew and desperately held onto would be over and completely forgotten.

During Jenna's last months, I watched as she wrestled with the realization that she was likely not going to beat cancer this fourth time. She always held out hope for God's healing, but what changed me forever was her desire to know Jesus more than for Him to heal her cancer. In theory, as a person following Christ, I knew this had to be the desire.

But how?

How do you actually believe and hold onto this when you are faced with the ever-present concept of death?

The difference I saw in Jenna when faced with this ongoing trial; she never lost sight of God's promises. She knew He would ultimately heal her, even if it wasn't on this Earth. She knew that the life He offered was so much more incredible than the life we could ever experience on our own. She knew that God was faithful and by trusting in Him through this unfathomable trial that she would receive the crown of everlasting life.

Jenna's faith was unshakable during these constant trials because she was anchored in His promises. She followed Jesus' example as He walked to the cross with the full awareness that He would die.

During her last week, Jenna knew that she would not be leaving the hospital again. In her last days, even though she didn't look like herself, she was more beautiful than I'd ever seen her. Her joy to see her Creator was infectious, and while our hearts were breaking with the awareness that we would be losing her, I couldn't help but trust in God's plan and His goodness because she had so fearlessly locked her eyes on Jesus.

In the hospital, we asked Jenna if she was scared. She confidently answered no. As each day passed, it was as if she became more at peace and excited about seeing Jesus. This made me question what I was holding onto in my life. What was I choosing to cling to over the excitement that I would one day see Jesus face to face? It was humbling and gut wrenching.

However, her incredible faith allowed me to wrestle with what my heart really wanted: this world or Heaven; earthly comforts or God's kingdom; my own plan or God's faithfulness.

After wrestling with these choices following Jenna's death, I found something I didn't expect. I found freedom. When I chose to let go of the things I was so desperately holding onto, there was comfort in knowing God's perfect plan would be fulfilled. Remarkably, it makes life a lot simpler. The question I am most frequently asked about Jenna's cancer and her death is *"If God is good, why would He not heal Jenna?"*

And I can hear Jenna say, *"Sweet friend, He did. He kept His promise."*

- *Ashley B.*

*"Blessed is the one who perseveres under trial because having stood the test, that person will receive the crown of life that the Lord has promised to those who love Him."*[1]

**James 1:12 (NIV)**

# Where it all started

## 05.03.15

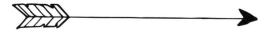

I'll be taking over the photography blog for a while, as God has me in this different phase of life right now, so it will be used as a place where people can come to find updates/know how to best pray for us. This first post I wrote before we knew all the things we know now, so I changed it a little, but wanted to keep some the same.

This is where it all started.

I was flipping through Isaiah this morning and came across this verse:

> *"I will turn the darkness into light before them*
> *and make the rough places smooth. These are the things*
> *I will do; I will not forsake them."* [1]
> **Isaiah 42:16 (NIV)**

I had flipped the page after seeing that, and God was telling me "Jenna, that is what I am doing here." I flipped back and wrote it down.

---

Time to back up and fill you in. Some of you may know, or may not, that I am an ovarian cancer survivor. I was diagnosed and treated in 2000 and then relapsed in 2002 and treated again. Any cancer survivor would tell you one of their greatest fears in life is relapse.

Having relapsed once already, about a year after I started following Jesus, I can say with everything I am, I am thankful for what that experience did to me.

I learned beyond a shadow of a doubt that the God I pledged my life to was everything He promised and more. He was faithful and present; He was my peace and strength. He provided every step of the way. He showed me in a very concrete way after that second battle with cancer that no matter what came my way in life; God was going to be enough.

---

Back up to a few weeks ago, I started getting waves of shooting pain in my lower abdomen. They weren't going anywhere so I shot an email to my nurse practitioner (NP) to keep her updated, and she ordered some labs and a couple ultrasounds.

This process happened very fast. I am a nurse in the hematology/oncology clinic that I was treated in 13 years ago. So, I work alongside some of my old doctors and nurse practitioners on a daily basis. It really is the best. I don't know if it is possible for someone to exist who loves his or her job more than I love mine.

There is a lab that we follow to track the tumor I had when I relapsed we knew it because it was increased, and that lab came back very slightly increased. Way less than we would expect it to be, but still a little increased. I was sitting at our triage desk when my NP told me over the phone.

I immediately started crying, but one of my sweet co-workers was there, and my NP came straight there after hanging up the phone. We talked through it, I calmed down, and made plans for the ultrasound.

Scott came with me to work the day of the ultrasound. The lady doing the ultrasound told me that she was the one that did my last ultrasound in 2005. What are the chances? The ultrasound of my abdomen looked good, which was good because I had radiation on my abdomen, so that's where we would have been expecting to see something.

I went back after I had a full bladder for the lower abdominal ultrasound. We did that ultrasound and within 5 minutes of it finishing were told that there was a mass between my remaining ovary and uterus.

The sweet radiologist brought me to a little room where we met with 2 of my NPs and one of our solid tumor doctors. I can't even describe to you how good it is in this situation to be surrounded by familiar faces and not strangers.

I'm being so detailed here, because these details have been the blessings God has given me so far in this situation to "*turn the darkness into light before them and make the rough places smooth.*"

They ordered an abdominal CT to rule out any spread in the upper abdomen, so we went out to the waiting room to re-register for that. While we were waiting, the doctor met us in there to check in. When I went back to get the CT, one of my co-workers came in to get the labs from the iv they placed.

Do you all see a theme of God putting friendly faces at every step here? I know this is a lot to read, but I'm telling you, God shows up in the details. The CT of the upper abdomen came back clear. I got multiple phone calls on our way home touching base and reporting findings. I know I'm an employee so I may be a bit biased, but there is no better care out there than there is at Cincinnati Children's. There's just not.

We went the next morning for the MRI at a satellite location. I was told I wouldn't hear anything until Monday (this was Friday), but that afternoon I got a call from my people giving me results. The MRI just confirmed with a slightly clearer picture what the ultrasound showed.

We wouldn't know much until we got in there to take it out and look at it under a microscope. Some of the characteristics came across as malignant, but the tumor marker was not as elevated as it should have been, so we really had no idea what it was.

I had surgery the following Thursday morning to get it taken out. That was another huge answer to prayer. I got the surgeon I wanted, and even with his packed schedule, I got in 3 days after I met with him. He even called me on my drive home from work to see if I had any questions.

I know God does not allow His people to walk head first into storms alone and without reason. He is going to be my ever-present comfort and peace in this, and He will use it so the people around me can see Him clearly. I have already had people remark about "my strength," and I want it to be known that it is not me. God is my rock, and without Him, I know this situation would be more than I could bear. The peace I've been experiencing throughout all of this is witness enough to His power and goodness.

I have always wondered what my reaction would be to facing this again. It is still one of my worst nightmares, but that's the thing about God, He is so much bigger than any circumstance we face.

We will be praying around the clock over here for benign results, but even if we don't get those results, I know the God who holds my life in His hands. And that makes every difference.

Thanks for hanging in here if you did. I am being very thorough because when things feel hard, it is so comforting to look back at how God has already shown up to be reminded that He is at work.

———

*"I will turn the darkness into light before them and make the rough places smooth. These are the things I will do; I will not forsake them."* [1]

**Isaiah 42:16 (NIV)**

# UNWAVERING FAITH

When reminiscing about Jenna, a floodgate of warm, positive memories flash back in my mind. The thought of seeing and working with Jenna always made me smile; it was a true honor to be her friend and work by her side.

During one shift, before finding out she had relapsed again, her doctor placed orders at our test referral center for Jenna to go and have her labs drawn after her shift. Since we were on the same team that day, we'd been conversing and speculating all afternoon about what could be going on.

Her doctor was also doing an education talk on cancer treatment for the nursing staff that evening, and Jenna and I decided that we'd go to test referral together first, then go to the talk, then walk to our parking garage together.

In my mind, I was cursing at God. I had a very bad feeling about Jenna's upcoming lab work, and I couldn't see how or why this was happening, potentially AGAIN. During this same time, I was experiencing very minor health issues that I was waiting on results for clarity and direction, but I begged Jesus to have my results come back negative and Jenna's to be favorable.

I pleaded.

Jenna and I walked to test referral; we sat in the waiting room. The entire time Jenna was positive, loving, and hopeful. Even though her situation was far scarier than mine, she asked for every detail about my medical scenario, selflessly putting my situation first.

Her faith was unwavering. I remember studying her face and was flabbergasted at how she could so purely exist in such a divine manner. In that moment, I knew Jesus Christ was real.

I could feel His love exuberating from Jenna. I realized how magnificently, but faithfully flawed we are. And I had a sense of peace, even though there were many outcomes I was uncertain of. I gained a greater appreciation, and a deeper sense of love for Jesus.

During times of happiness, sorrow, and confusion, I turn to prayer. I cried my entire commute and prayed the entire rosary for Jenna. I decided to text her to tell her that I was praying, not expecting a response. She then let me know that her lab results were elevated, and that she would be needing scans, and thanked me for praying.

My response was "*Always.*" {Which is part of a quote from Harry Potter that I am sure she noticed} From that moment on, I will always believe, I will always pray, and I will always continue to strive to know Jesus and uncover His teachings through ordinary events, as opposed to expecting His love to be seen only in extraordinary ways.

*- Kara B.*

# You've never failed

## 05.03.15

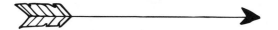

There is a song by Hillsong United that I told Scott I thought was written for me in this battle. My church is doing this series about being brave in storms; the timing is absolutely not a coincidence. You can't believe in God and believe in coincidence.

The song is called "Oceans." EVERY. SINGLE. WORD. is straight from God to my heart. The most meaningful to me is *"Where feet may fail and fear surrounds me, you've never failed, and you won't start now."*

I mean, come on. Having walked through this battle twice now, knowing that He has been faithful, it's like He's telling me over and over, *"I've got you, Jenna."*

This song was played the week before this all started on day 2 of the pain. I sang it with tears in my eyes knowing something was not right.

There are words that say, *"Spirit lead me where my trust is without borders, let me walk upon the waters wherever you would call me. Take me deeper than my feet could ever wander, and my faith will be made stronger in the presence of my Savior."* [1] I sang those words that day knowing those are scary words to say to God.

And here is where I stand now. I am going to walk forward on waters that are stormy, but I will keep my eyes above those waves on Jesus Himself. He has a plan for this. I want Him to be lifted so high in this journey. I want people to see His goodness in this. I know that He doesn't leave us in these storms on our own. When Peter walked on water, the minute he took his eyes off of Jesus and focused on the waves, he started to sink. But Jesus IMMEDIATELY reached His hand down to catch him. Even on the days I focus more on the waves than Jesus, I know His hand is waiting to pull me back up.[3]

Alright, I had to start there, time for updating. After my MRI that Friday, I knew that the mass was looking malignant. Like I said, my church is doing this series, and that Saturday before my surgery the sermon was about storms specifically. Chuck, one of the pastors, specifically said, *"Maybe your storm is a diagnosis."* Every word specifically tailored to my heart. Reminding me He is faithful and present.

I worked my last shift on that Monday, and got to meet with the surgeon during my lunch break. He was going to be going out of town soon, but managed to squeeze me into a packed schedule. I know I've mentioned it before, but I work in the same clinic that I was treated in, and will be treated in again, so all day I had everyone I needed for questions right at my fingertips. My job is such a blessing in so many ways.

Scott and I arrived for surgery on Thursday morning. We checked in at the front desk and they asked, "Just the 3 of you?" assuming Scott and I were bringing our kid for surgery. Funny things like that happen when you're 28, going to a children's hospital.

My friend Lauren was working in pre-op that day so I got to see her, and even my anesthesiologist was a friend of a friend and also a believer that would be praying for me. Do you all see how God's not leaving a detail to chance here? He is so good.

The surgery lasted about 3 hours, and the surgeon got the tumor out. It didn't come out easy, but piece by piece, since it was stuck up to surrounding tissue. They told me it looked like the same tumor from 2000 and 2002, but that we had to wait for pathology to have final answers.

Recovery could not have gone better. We left the hospital the morning of the 4$^{th}$ day, and had friends who brought breakfast that walked out with us. I had sweet friends visit from Lexington, sweet co-workers that came up to the room; the encouragement was so great.

My doctor called me the following day with the pathology report, telling me that it was in fact the same cancer. I knew that, but hearing it confirmed was not easy. Scott was out when I got the call, but man, God showed up.

Immediately upon hanging up the phone, I had a notice from the app my church is using for our brave journey saying I had a message. I opened it up and it was Isaiah 43:2.

First of all. Isaiah is my favorite, second, this is my favorite verse in Isaiah. Third, it was exactly what I needed to hear.

Not a coincidence. God was immediately telling me, *"Don't worry Jenna, I'm carrying you through this, I've got you."* He has not left me to face this alone even for a minute. Ya'll, He is everything we need. He is faithful to carry you through every valley, every battle. And not just for people "like me." For all of us.

Thank you all for reading if you still are. I need to have all these details recorded because I don't want to forget.

*"When you pass through the waters, I will be with you;*

*and when you pass through the rivers,*

*they will not sweep over you.*

*When you walk through the fire, you will not be burned;*

*the flames will not set you ablaze."* [2]

**Isaiah 43:2 (NIV)**

# OVERFLOWING HOPE

I always knew God was good, but I struggled to really hold on to that as I received updates about Jenna through those months she fought cancer. I'd never lost anyone important to me before Jenna, and I'd never been close to something like this, something that made me realize how painful and unfair life could really be. I was pushed into my Bible to find hope and healing and to remind myself why God was good and loving. But the most encouragement, I think, came from Jenna.

She had this really amazing way of glorifying God even in the hard times. The fact that she held on to God and glorified Him and was excited about Him even in the pain, strengthened me as I witnessed her taking on her greatest trial with more grace, strength, and hope than is humanly possible. I believe she got that kind of spirit from God, and boy, I pray that someday I can have that same kind of strength. I aspire to have a spirit as lovely and hopeful as hers.

Jenna took a time that would break the strongest people and turned it into an opportunity to magnify the goodness of God. No matter how dark it got, I only saw that she shined the light brighter to the point that through her death, she only showed me how much greater God was. I saw her crave God, and I saw her hope for healing and her hope for Jesus. I saw her hope in a promise that she would be with God and experiencing a life with more fullness and love, and that ultimately, her life would be a testament to His goodness and faithfulness no matter what happened.

Because of Jenna's hope, my view of God only turned more loving, more graceful, and more caring. Her intense love for Him made me crave Him all the more. She inspires me to value God more than anything in my life. He is the only part of my life that will last, the only one I will get to take with me in death, and the one who will be with me on the other side. Investing in my love for God is the best thing I can do with my life. She did that, and because of it I saw Life overflow, especially in the midst of death.

There is so much Life with God, and death really doesn't overcome that. It's an everlasting Life that can pour out of us, like it did with Jenna. It's still pouring out, and I am so encouraged because death still hasn't overcome her and never will. She's with God and because of that, I know she's more alive now than ever before.

*- Sarah E.*

# Treatment plans

## 05.03.15

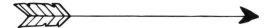

Last Wednesday we went to the clinic to talk treatment plans with my new team. I had to get a new Nurse Practitioner (NP) and a care manager, all that. But again, I work in this clinic, so even the new faces were familiar faces. It makes a huge difference.

We are going to proceed with 6 cycles of chemotherapy. Before we start that, Scott and I decided to freeze some eggs in case treatment jeopardizes our fertility in the future.

We were given 2 weeks to get that taken care of before treatment would start. I went in prepared for this plan. I would have felt uncomfortable doing nothing about this. There are most likely residual cells left over because of how stuck the tumor was to surrounding tissue, so I want to do everything we need to do to kill those.

Radiation is still on the table as an option, but we haven't decided about that yet. Before I left, my sweet co-workers hunted me down to give me a care basket and hugs.

Scott and I met with the fertility people on Friday. We walked into that appointment and were told that the only cost we'd have to pay was a yearly storage fee. Kind of pricey, but doable. We had to get in to get the ball rolling to be done in time for treatment to start. There are a lot of extra charges in there. I know that we're getting an amazing deal because this is a cancer related thing, but we are just not in a spot financially to swing the costs.

Over this weekend we're making hard choices about whether to move forward or not. This has sadly been the most stressful thing we've faced. There are a lot of unanswered questions on the table that would help us make this decision, but because of timing we have to make that decision without knowing solid answers.

We went to church yesterday, again still in this Brave journey. The first song they played is one of the most meaningful songs to me. It's called "You Are Mine," and basically it is a conversation between someone struggling and God. The chorus is adapted from my favorite verse, Isaiah 43:2.

> "When you walk through the water, I will be with you
> When you pass through the river, the waves will not overtake you
> When you walk on the fire, the flames they will not touch you
> You are mine, you are mine, you are mine." [1]

I mean, come on. Could God be any clearer? Yes, He could, because the next song they played was "How He Loves" by David Crowder. Another song that cuts right to my heart.

During the service Brian said, "If we bring all our resources and still don't have enough, we can bravely go forward and trust in Him." Are you kidding me? It's like God was sitting there with me saying, "I've got this." He knows that this decision is a struggle financially. I know without a shadow of a doubt that if we walk forward with this process, that He will provide the means to pay for it.

They ended the service with "Oceans." I am one hundred percent sure that this song was written for my heart. I won't repeat lyrics, because I wrote them in the last post.

How blessed am I with my community, with a God that speaks so directly and tenderly to my heart, with a church that seems to be right on target with a huge storm in my life?

God is good.

That is it for now. Tomorrow Scott and I will make a decision about proceeding with egg retrieval, and if we go forward, I will probably be ridiculously over emotional due to all the hormones, but God will show up in that too, I don't doubt.

For specific prayers moving forward, pray for us financially, that God would provide. Pray for continued peace. He has flooded me with peace every step of the way so far, and it is so crazy and awesome. Philippians 4:7 says, *"And the peace of God, which surpasses all understanding, will guard your hearts and your minds in Christ Jesus."*[2] I believe all Scripture is God breathed and this is one of the promises that He has flooded my life with specifically in this process. Be praying for the doctors specifically in the area of decisions about radiation.

Thanks you all; I know three posts in one day is a lot but I wanted to get everything down before things got too crazy. Thanks for tracking along.

———

*"And the peace of God, which surpasses all understanding, will guard your hearts and your minds in Christ Jesus."*[2]

**Philippians 4:7**

# REVELATION SONG

The first night I hung out with Jenna, a large group of us (who met through Young Life) went out to the movies. The movie choice: *Saw*. Jenna and I both really hate horror films, so we probably watched a whole 10 minutes of the ridiculousness. However, we both had such a desire to hang out with people that it almost didn't matter what the plan was or what the movie was, because we would be there—with all of our people.

After the movie was over, I remember getting Jenna's phone number and her saying that her last name was "Gilfedder," and that she couldn't wait to be married to have a new last name. Over time, Gilfedder morphed into so many nicknames that it really became somewhat of a silly identity for college-Jenna. Although, it isn't your name that will define your identity, but rather, it is your character. Jenna bestowed the best characteristics we all wish to have.

She was energetic, joyful, compassionate, servant-hearted, and faithful beyond measure. Faithfulness is the one characteristic I saw consistently maturing in Jenna over the last 12 years. Faithful to her friends, in all phases of life; to her Young Life team amidst change and adversity; to high school students, despite their poor decision-making and sometimes seemingly fruitless lives; to getting her nursing degree, even when her advisors told her she probably would not; faithful to Scott through a long-distance relationship and questions about what their future home would look like as they opened it up to energetic, destructive teenagers.

Jenna was a committed friend who would drive hours just to be at a birthday party because she valued and loved them so much. However, Jenna's utmost faithfulness was to the Lord.

When I think of Jenna's life, I immediately think of her unwavering commitment to God. A faithfulness that was rooted, confident, and steadfast. It is no surprise that when Jenna's cancer returned, her posture about the Lord remained unchanged. She was faithful to the Lord's good work in her life and in others. Faithful to His plan, even when she had received hard news. And most admirably—faithful to sharing the Good News of Christ.

Jenna's demeanor was always gracious, subtle, and affectionate (and thank goodness for that because we have so many loud and crazy friends!), so the way she spoke so fondly of the Lord and that He was good above all things made you want to lean in and learn more.

It is without doubt, that the last two years of Jenna enduring cancer allowed me to grow closer to the Lord and recognize the preeminence of His life over *all* things more than I ever had before.

Our friends always joke that Jenna was everyone's favorite friend, which is true, because she was wonderful in so many ways. But, I believe that her steadfast devotion to the Lord and her deep love for people were the most contagious characteristics that allowed her to be a radiant light in a clouded and sometimes horrifying world.

Right before Jenna's last week I had a dream of our friends crowded around her bed singing "Revelation Song"[1] and worshiping the Lord in His goodness and holiness. So that is what we did. We blubbered through tears and forgotten lyrics as we ushered our faithful friend home to Jesus. I believe wholeheartedly that she was greeted by the Lord with Him saying, "Well done, my good and faithful servant," because that defines the identity of our sweet, dear Jenna.

- *Julie M.*

# What a week

## 05.08.15

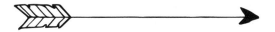

W hat a week. A whole lot has happened since posting everything last Sunday. Scott and I have had to make a lot of hard decisions in the past few days. A lot of decisions we didn't see coming.

The last we left you all with, we were planning on going forward with egg preservation, but we could not afford it. Some of our best friends here in Batesville put together a "GoFundMe" page, and on Sunday night they showed it to us. The upfront costs had been covered ... in 24 hours.

And that doesn't even include sweet friends that reached out to us wanting to give.

Scott and I struggled a lot with this, because it is very hard to receive. But the weight that it took off of our backs was so incredible. We felt like we could make this decision based on what we wanted to do, and not on our finances. God is showing us so much in this process, and one of those things is to learn how to let people serve us and love us.

The ways God has showed up through the people in our lives has been more than we even can put to words. Scott and I made a meal for the first time tonight—I had surgery 15 days ago.

Whether it be financially, with a home-cooked meal, or even just people showing up to do life with us, pass time with us, we have been so loved, and we could not be more thankful.

Oh man. That being said, these past few days have been HARD. On Monday, we went to the fertility office to get an ultrasound and some labs so we could start taking the stimulation meds. On the ultrasound, there was a large cyst on my ovary, which was not optimal, but we were going to move forward because we didn't have time to wait. Then my labs came back going in the wrong direction. So if I had started the medications, they would not have worked the way they would need to.

We started having some hard conversations with the team. There were a lot of things standing in our way. The shots that would stimulate egg growth, we believe would also stimulate tumor growth. The retrieval process would be going through areas with residual cancer cells, which could introduce those cells to all the areas the needle passed into and out of. The presence of the cysts would limit the amount of eggs we could retrieve to 2-3 eggs.

We also found out that radiation is looking like something that will happen, and that would count the uterus out as far as carrying a pregnancy goes.

Like I said, a lot. Scott and I had to have a lot of conversations about what different options we have of having biological kids, how we feel about adopting, all things we were not super prepared to have with such a short time frame to answer. I wanted so badly to be pregnant one day.

I was flipping through Instagram the other day and I saw a quote that I needed. It said, *"God never denies our hearts desire except to give us something better."[1]* I don't know who said that, *but I know God's heart. I know He loves us, and I know He is good.*

So while it may look like a lot of closed doors, I know He cares deeply about these situations, and He has a plan, and really that is all I need to move forward. It doesn't make it less hard, but it gives me peace in the difficulty.

I stumbled across 1 Samuel 12:16, which says,

> *"Now therefore stand still and see this great thing that the Lord will do before your eyes."* [2]

I wrote it down, because in these past few weeks there has been no accidental stumbling over verses. If they come across my path, they have been the very breath of God to me. I know I can rest in Him with every single problem that has come our way. Is it still hard? Yes. Absolutely. But I was talking with Scott, and can honestly say, I am thankful. The ways that trials open my eyes and connect me to God, it is worth the struggle. I have felt so connected to Him with every single step. That connection is worth more than any season of blessing in our lives. There is no area of my life right now where I feel I am living on the surface. That is a blessing.

This past Thursday after the decision was made about to not proceed with the egg retrieval, we went to the Brave experience. Our church is on a journey, which I've written about a lot already. They have a prayer experience set up, where you go and put on headphones that guide you through rooms set up for you to meet with God. Rooms that set you up to face the storms in your life, and set you up to be at the feet of Jesus.

Scott and I had the chance to sit on sailboats, to literally walk through a room that was set up to look like you were walking through stormy waters. All the while you are listening to prompts that pointed to God, to wrestle with the hard things in life, to ask God hard questions. Perfect timing yet again.

At the end, you can have someone pray for you, and Scott and I both knew this was something we couldn't pass up. The sweet girl who prayed for us, we felt, was sort of casting a vision over us. I knew that God was giving her words to say to us.

What stood out to me was that *this story was very important to God. Our specific story was important to Him. That He didn't want this for us. But that He will use it.* Words that I needed to hear so badly.

I know this is getting long, thanks for sticking with me, if you have. After a long day of tests at the hospital to make sure my body can handle the chemotherapy I'll be getting, we talked with our doctor and made a plan to go ahead and get a line placed and start chemo Monday or Tuesday next week. I joked with Scott today that we've been so busy battling all of the other issues that we haven't really processed the reality of this. So this weekend will hopefully be filled with a lot of rest and fun and hearing from God. I know that the last will at least be true. He is so faithful.

Lastly, if you are someone who has donated to our "GoFundMe" page, know that from the **bottom of our hearts**, we could not thank you enough. It means so much to be able to walk into this without worrying about paying the bills. Our deductible starts over again at the end of this month, so bills will be coming.

We are praying about what to do if there is excess, because a lot of people gave money specifically for fertility. We want that excess to go to building our family, so whatever that looks like, be it surrogacy, adoption, wherever God leads us as far as family, know that you are a huge help to us.

Also, thank you to those of you who have shared with us how God was leading you to pray for us. You know who you are, and your words have been exactly what we've needed to hear. He truly has blessed us beyond what we deserve with you all in our lives.

*"Worship despite circumstances; He is always at work."*
**A note from Jenna next to Acts 16:25**

*"About midnight Paul and Silas were praying and singing hymns to God, and the prisoners were listening to them,"* [3]
**Acts 16:25**

# FACING INFERTILITY

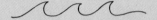

For 7 years we waited, and for 7 years our faith was tested through relentless heartbreaks and disappointments. As we faced our battle, Jenna was a faithful friend and prayer warrior for our family.

Jenna though, had her own terrible realities to face. While receiving treatment for her cancer, major concerns were brought up about the effects this would have on her eggs and her ability to have children. As hard as this must have been to hear, she decided it would be best to try and preserve as many eggs as possible by freezing them, and that required many of the same medications and procedures that were also a part of our IVF treatments.

These medications can be thousands of dollars for just one round of IVF, and because she was a cancer patient, Jenna was able to receive them for significantly less.

When she found out she would be unable to freeze her eggs, she called and offered to give me her unused medication for our procedure. While she was fighting for her life, she was still thinking of others and looking to their needs, rather than focusing on her own.

To find out that you'd be unable to have children is devastating news, yet Jenna thought of how she could use her change in circumstance to bless others.

To see how Jenna selflessly loved others during her trial

changed the way that I faced my own. To not focus solely on my own challenges but to always be looking for ways to love and bless others in the midst of them. This gave me the ability to change my outlook on life.

Jenna encouraged us to keep the faith through bad news and disappointments; to strive to be more like Jesus and love others, rather than focus on ourselves and our challenges.

I'm so thankful for the way Jenna faced her trials and showed us Jesus in her suffering. It changed the way we faced our own suffering.

In August of 2017, we welcomed our son Theo into the world. We wish so much that she was here to snuggle sweet Theo and see that her faithful prayers were answered by our gracious God.

*- Anne W.*

# First chemo down

## 05.21.15

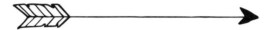

This first chemo went so well. Thank you so much for those of you that were praying about it. We went in last Wednesday to get a port placed and to get admitted. We waited all day in pre-op, but got in at the last second.

The port placement went well with no collapsed lungs this time! The first chemo consisted of a 4-day inpatient stay (3 days of chemo, 1 day of getting hydration and a shot to keep my counts from dropping too low).

I had all kinds of sweet visitors bearing non-hospital food, coffee for Scott, press-n-seal so that I could shower without getting my port dressing too wet, bags full of Target gifts, my favorite salad from Lexington.

Also, our friend Sean took some photos of us with my camera the day before we went in for chemo. They'll be so good to have when I don't feel like I look like myself at all. We love them so much!

Seriously to all of you who visited while at work, who drove from Lexington and Batesville, who visited while your kiddo was in the hospital, we appreciate you all so much. Time went so quickly because of you.

Scott found out that family members can use a gym and get massages while in the hospital, and that made his stay more bearable. I walked around with my IV pole, visiting my friends at work and giving tours to my visiting friends.

No nausea or vomiting. Praise the Lord. Thanks to a lot of medication and a lot of you all praying, that was not an issue. I keep saying how the first couple times I went through this I never got sick, never needed blood products, etc. I think when you're not a teenager anymore your body doesn't always respond the same, so I am very thankful for round 1 to be finished without getting sick.

I will tell you that recovery was definitely the same at home. The thing (other than losing hair) that I hated the most was post-chemo. For those of you that have been there, you know that you kind of check out for a few days. It's hard to explain but I will try my best.

For 2-3 days after we got home, sitting up on the couch from a laying position felt like I may as well have run a marathon. Maybe worse. I've never run a marathon. Even in responding to Scott, I could not muster enough energy to respond with any kind of enthusiasm or inflection. I felt like I just checked out from life for a few days. I remember thinking "I will never complain about being tired again when I get better."

Today, I'm typing this and my counts are looking good and I still am not back to my normal, but I am showered and wearing real clothes and that is enough reason to be thankful.

One thing I did not expect was a lot of skin pain. It was very tender to touch and almost felt bruised around my neck, sides, and upper back. I'd take it any day over nausea and vomiting, but it was not fun.

I have been reading a book given to me by some of my co-workers called *Every Bitter Thing is Sweet* by Sara Hagerty. It is so good. The author wrote about the hard things in her life and how she knew God deeply out of those things. So much good truth. I want to just quote the entire book. But I'll settle with just one for now.

> *"Fear loses oxygen when every moment suspends itself under the purpose of bringing Him glory, of knowing His name and His nature. Sometimes, instead of leading us up and out of those very fears, big and small, He lets us live them. He gives us over to them. Because it's in this giving over to our fears that we find the perfect love that frees us from them. Forever."* [1]

I think the difference between this time with cancer and the second time with cancer is that it isn't so much about the cancer this time. This time it's about what God is doing. Where He is leading Scott and me. Where we will end up after this with our faith. How He is going to use this. Yes, the path is not fun. It is not what I would have chosen, not what Scott would have chosen. But if we know God better at the end of this, *isn't it worth it?*

I read a blog post recently about how, as Christians, we are still striving so much for comfort. We strive for comfort when we follow a God that says, *"take up your cross and follow me"* [2]—a good God who loves us and has the best in mind for us.

Who cares if we have it "hard" in this life when we have eternity stretched out before us? This life is the only chance that we have to have faith, to make an impact. I know me, and I am not one to grow when things are comfortable and easy. So, yes, I'll take this hard road ahead if it means spiritual growth, if it means Jesus gets lifted high, and the people around me can see Him more clearly.

I'll have all the comfort I need in eternity one day. He is good.

One last thing. I was listening to a mix I made on iTunes the day before we went in for chemo. I had thrown a random song on there that I hadn't heard in years. I had no memory about what the words were when I added it to the playlist. It was so incredibly perfect.

*I have unanswered prayers*
*I have trouble I wish wasn't there*
*And I have asked a thousand ways*
*That you would take my pain away*
*You would take my pain away*

*I am trying to understand*
*How to walk this weary land*
*Make straight the paths that crooked lie*
*Oh Lord, before these feet of mine*
*Oh Lord, before these feet of mine*

*When my world is shaking, heaven stands*
*When my heart is breaking I never leave your hands*

*When you walked upon the earth*
*You healed the broken, lost and hurt*
*I know you hate to see me cry*
*One day you will set all things right*
*Yeah, one day you will set all things right*

*When my world is shaking, heaven stands*
*When my heart is breaking I never leave your hands* [3]

Your Hands
**JJ Heller**

# FRENCH BRAIDS

I was young. 19. I had just finished my first year of college and God was starting to stir in me a new way of hearing Him. Up to that point I really only looked for signs from Him. Outside-of-me kinda stuff. But that summer He started working within, speaking within.

It was June and I had no idea that I'd be making big changes in my life based on these stirrings and speakings. But first, Young Life camp. I was invited to be a guest leader at a week of camp.

Lucky me! Full time leaders had been building relationships with students for years and I got to show up for a week of fun and do my best to help.

I ended up leading Jenna's cabin.

Oh Jenna. Pure sunshine. Maybe 15 at the time.

Though a leader, I was still nervous that I didn't really know anyone. Jenna treated me like we'd been friends for years. Adopted me. She stood out. I honestly don't remember anyone else but her. Her and her sunshine.

Midway through the week she asked me to French braid her hair. Sitting on the dusty, low-pile carpet floor of our cabin I prepped to braid. Just as I grabbed a strand of her hair she jumped up and said, *"OH WAIT! Let me get my clips or my hair will fall off!"*

"WHAT?!" I exclaimed. So confused, so shocked.

She laughed. "I had cancer and my hair hasn't grown back yet. It's like peach fuzz. This is a wig!"

She laughed. I laughed.

Amazed at her unrelenting joy, I braided her hair as she told me the rest of that story.

I will forever remember that moment—listening, knees on the hard floor, the smells of summer camp, timidly braiding, curiously considering the texture of the hair and being careful not to pull too hard.

This, the beginning of a sweet gift of a friendship and my deep admiration of Jenna. That week I heard clearly from God, sitting next to Jenna at the final camp gathering. No big signs, just quiet words that resonated within.

"I am faithful," He said.

Not in a "Look back and see how faithful I have been" kind of way. But instead, a forward-looking "hold onto your butts" kind of way. Not, "See? I've been faithful." But "I am faithful ... (now hold on)."

Of course, at the time, I was simply thinking about what that meant for the summer ahead. What it meant in my OWN life. Not 15 years ahead. Not in my friendship with Jenna.

But 15 years ahead I'd be weeping in both sorrow and gratitude at Jenna's memorial service.

Sorrow for the loss. Gratitude that Jenna stood out and adopted me. Trying to muster up a fraction of her joy. Remembering her pure sunshine. Remembering those words I heard in her company.

"I am faithful ... (now hold on)."

*- Andrea V.*

# Hair loss & truth

## 06.05.15

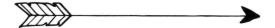

There is a funny thing that happens in between cycles of chemotherapy. After the first week of fatigue, you start to get some energy back. Then you start to feel like a normal person again.

Specific to this time after the first cycle of chemo, you still have a full head of hair. Other than a port that bothers you when you move a certain way, you may as well be as healthy as anyone.

Now I have a big break. Technically round two of chemo should have happened yesterday, but today I got home from a week of family vacation, and on Monday Scott and I leave for our favorite week of the year:

Young Life camp!

The only thing that really disrupts your feeling like a normal person again is getting labs drawn regularly, and you start shedding. It starts out as a few more hairs in your brush, and next thing you know you're sitting outside at dinner on vacation and you see a clump of hair fly over the table in front of your 2-year-old nephew.

If you're following along on our journey here, you know this isn't my first rodeo. I've done the hair falling out thing before. Last time it happened, I was a teenager. I was in high school. I cared A LOT about losing my hair.

This time is different in that I don't know that I'll wear a wig all the time. Last time I didn't ever take it off. Nobody saw me without it. Except for one time I was in the car with a friend and got rear-ended and my wig flew off. It made for a great story later.

So here I am facing a week of camp, wondering whether or not to just shave it all off and wear cute headbands all week, or to keep it and shed all over the place. I'm struggling with this decision more than I thought. I know it's just hair. I know this is trivial compared to the greater thing at work here. But this is hard.

It doesn't help that my sweet friend Donielle gave me the cutest short bob ever. I will always have this haircut when it grows back.

Those are all my thoughts on hair. Last time I wrote, I shared that I was reading a book called *Every Bitter Thing is Sweet* by Sara Hagerty. This book could have been written from my heart. Our circumstances aren't all the same, but the truths about growth and closeness to the Lord through the hardships are. I made a habit of circling page numbers when I wanted to go back and look at specific quotes. I want to share all of them, as I've said, but I won't do that to you. Just go read it, you won't be disappointed.

She writes, *"Every single ache, large and small, had a response from a God who put on skin so that I might know His scent and feel His hands and live in a nearness that would forever keep me coming back to sit at His feet."* [1]

Oh man. I would call cancer the large ache, and hair loss the small. It is a good reminder for me that He is there drawing me to Him. Even in this inward battle I am having with not having hair, He is saying "Bring it to me," and He is more than enough to meet me there.

That is it for now. Scott and I have a hard choice to make regarding radiation over this next week, so we ask for your prayers that God would lead us down whatever road He wants us. Love you all, thank you so much for reading and praying for us. God is big, and He is moving.

——

*"Every single ache, large and small, had a response*
*from a God who put on skin so that I might know*
*His scent and feel His hands and live in a nearness that*
*would forever keep me coming back to sit at His feet."* [1]

**Sara Hagerty**

# Dear Lord,

## - ROOTS TO GROW DEEP -

## 06.16.15

Father,

It has been 14 years, you have been so faithful. I thank you for holding tightly to me, Lord. I pray I would never wander away from you. I thank you for using me in the lives of the girls at the high school. I ask you to give them roots. I pray you would move in their lives in a way that causes them to trust you and cling to you with all they have. Help me to lead them well.

I give you Scott, I thank you for him. Bless our marriage, Lord. Bring us on the same page as far as radiation goes. Work on our hearts if you want us to adopt, Lord. Be at work and open our eyes and ears to see you working and hear from you. I praise you that the PET scan looked good. I love you, Lord. In your Son's name I give you everything. Amen.

*But when Jesus heard it he said, "This illness
does not lead to death. It is for the glory of God,
so that the Son of God may be glorified through it."* [1]

**John 11:4**

# THROUGH MY FEARS

I did not know Jenna as long or as well as I would have liked, but that doesn't mean her life has not affected my walk with Jesus. Jenna was in the middle of a terrifying situation and yet, she showed no sign of fear. She wholeheartedly believed every promise God made to her and because of this, lived life rooted in that belief.

She wanted to be healed, but also couldn't wait to see the face of the One who saved her and was everything to her. She comforted those she loved and was leaving behind, knowing that she would see them again. She wanted her celebration of life service to point everyone to Jesus. Her bold faith was extraordinary.

Because of Jenna, I want to live out my faith boldly; outside of my comfort zone. God is much bigger than my fears and inadequacies. He calls me to fully rely on Him in everything I do without a self-made safety net. I know this won't be easy because I am not a risk taker. But it is in those moments I think of Jenna and remember, He is with me, just as He was with her.

*– Susan B.*

# Dear Lord,

## - PRESENT IN THE SORROWS -

## 06.23.15

Jesus,

I thank you for the book loaned to me by Susan that reminded me of the importance of mourning; of getting it out. There are times I can easily praise you in this trial and then there are times where I am just sad.

But you don't leave me there alone.

I get sad when I look in the mirror and am bald for a third time. I'm sad when my upcoming 13-year cancer free gets dwindled right back down to 0. I'm sad that Scott and I have to choose between two awful options with radiation.

I'm sad I won't ever wait on a pregnancy test with joyful expectation. I'm sad that chemo knocks me out, feeling tired and in pain for a few days at a time. I'm sad Scott has to have a bald wife. I'm sad I can't have a ponytail. I'm sad life isn't as carefree as it was in the photos I looked through today.

BUT.

You are good, Lord. I know this to my core, and for that I thank you. That doesn't fix my long list of disappointments, but it does direct my focus to the One who doesn't leave me to muddle through them alone. I thank you for being my ever-present help. I thank you for your peace, given without limit.

Jesus, mend my broken areas and mold me to look more like you. Help me to structure my days around you, Lord. Go before me each day and open my eyes to see where you are moving. In your perfect and good name I give myself to you.

Amen.

———

*"Now therefore stand still and see this great*
*thing that the Lord will do before your eyes."* [1]
**1 Samuel 12:16**

# MUDDY SHOES &
# SORE MUSCLES

I had two thoughts when I first met Jenna. One, *this girl is going to need me to show her the ropes.* And two, *is this girl for real?* I had never met anyone like Jenna before, and I mistook her for being naïve.

She seemed to lock in on one idea and obsess over it—like New Jersey bagels or the Yankees or Red Lobster's cheddar biscuits. She was quiet and soft-spoken, almost childlike in her approach to life. She was sweet. Sweeter than sweet. So sweet, in fact, that people would ask me for many years after that, "Is she for real?" For those of us who knew her well, we knew that there was something set apart about Jenna from the beginning. She was different.

What I did not immediately recognize was how genuine Jenna's faith in the Lord was. It was clear to see that she was meek. And that she was humble. But she was also incredibly wise.

Where I boasted with confidence in my abilities, she humbly spoke with confidence in the Lord's promises. I soon realized that she was not going to need me to help her learn how to lead high school girls. I was going to need to learn how to shine like Jenna did for the Lord.

For several years, Stephanie, Jenna, and I were the

female Young Life leaders at a local High School. One summer at Rockbridge (A Young Life camp in Virginia), we graciously bowed out of the bike ride when they announced that camp was too full and some cabins would have to skip. Our cabin of girls rejoiced that we had spared them from trekking through the woods on mountain bikes and being sore for the next two days.

The following summer, the returning campers began to complain and had convinced Stephanie and I that we should once again, skip the bike ride altogether.

But it was Jenna, the least athletically enthused leader of us all, who insisted that we complete the outing as a cabin. She said that we needed to challenge the girls to do something they didn't want to do and didn't think they could do. And she was right. That bike trip was so worth it—muddy shoes and sore muscles included.

The girls felt accomplished and proud of themselves. We laughed and had lasting jokes to share about our time in the woods. It brought us closer together as a cabin, allowing them to trust that their leaders would not push them beyond their abilities.

Jenna knew that the bike trip paralleled a trusting relationship with the Lord. God was working in the hearts of each of those girls that week, and she knew the bike trip was one piece of the puzzle where we should not stand in the way of His work.

This is one of my least significant memories of all the wonderful times I spent with Jenna. From our wedding days, to road trips, and years of Bible study together, we shared so many incredible moments.

Yet that simple picture of Jenna at Young Life camp

speaks volumes about who she was. She could have easily given in to temptation, because we all know she didn't want to ride a mountain bike. But she sacrificed her own comfort for the growth of others.

That was the thing about Jenna: she pushed you towards the Lord without ever being pushy. Just being near her was a challenge to your own faith, yet she so gracefully lived her life with a sweet and caring disposition.

When we lost Jenna, we lost a wise woman who sought out the Lord's guidance in everything. I lost one of my best friends, someone that I counted on to point me to Christ by the way she lived and loved.

And in her death, we have gained one thing: a faith more like Jenna's. Because you couldn't see her so gracefully accept death and so hopefully embrace Heaven and not have your own faith grow.

When you try to make sense of why Jenna is gone from this life, the only possible answer is that even though she was glorifying the Lord so much with her life, she glorified Him even more with her death.

I know that when people die, it's common to overlook their shortcomings and memorialize their character by slightly exaggerating. This is not the case with Jenna. We are not reading exaggerated descriptions of her character and tall tales of her experiences. The very things that have been said about Jenna since her death are the very things that were said about her during her life. *Was this girl for real?* She absolutely was. The kind of real that the Lord can produce in each of us, if we are willing.

*- Katie H.*

# 2nd chemo down
# & Young Life camp

## 06.23.15

Chemo number two is over and done. A whole lot has happened since my last update. I'll try a quick recap.

I was debating on whether or not to shave my hair before Young Life (YL) camp. My choice became very clear when I was filling up a lint roller every 5 minutes with my shedding hair. Nobody wants to deal with that at YL camp.

I had Scott shave it off for me, but before I let him, I wanted to brush through it. You all, I hadn't brushed my hair in over a week before that. Part of that was my super easy to deal with haircut, but the other part was that it would have been a full brush with every swoop.

I wouldn't even rub a towel through it to dry it. I just patted it down. One thing that is not shared very much is that when hair falls out, it hurts. It does not feel good to rub, so pat-dry it was.

You can imagine after a week of no brushing and patting it dry, running a brush through it was pretty wonderful. It was tender for sure, but so nice. I filled up my brush about 8 times overflowing with hair and then decided to just pull out all that I could. I made a very sizeable pile in the trash can, and then let Scott do his thing.

For those wondering, this does not hurt, and is kind of nice when you've been tip-toeing around your hair for over a week. Scott was so sweet and made the otherwise sad process very light. He made sad noises with every swoop of the clippers. It was pretty adorable.

On to camp!

Scott and I boarded a packed Greyhound bus full of teenagers the next morning and headed to Rockbridge, the Young Life camp in Virginia.

Rockbridge is a magical place, y'all. What a great first week of not having hair. It is literally life as it's meant to be. I didn't even have time to focus on my new lack of hair. I got to live life intentionally with an entire cabin of teenagers and talk to them about a God who loves them and gave His life for them.

How often do we get to slow down and have deep, intentional conversations? I love camp because it creates that environment with ease. They got to hear why life is so hard and messed up, and they got to see Jesus clearly, the Jesus who came to offer them real life. I can't think of a greater privilege God has given me than being able to lead Young Life, and that is always at its peak during summer camp.

One thing I noticed while at camp is that prior to hair loss, I felt like God gave me this story that was just bottled up inside, and unless you know me personally, you wouldn't know to ask. I think losing your hair is a great way to share your story. People are more likely to approach you and ask. I am not one to walk up to a stranger and tell them my whole life. God knows this about me. So a silver lining of hair loss is that it makes you a walking testimony.

I'm making all of this sound easy, and I don't want that to be what you leave with. I have days where I look in the mirror and think to myself,

*"Really? We're doing this again?"*

It is frustrating. It is frustrating that in a couple weeks I could have said I was 13 years cancer-free and now we are restarting from scratch.

It's frustrating that after losing my hair twice, I lost it after getting it to record length.

It's frustrating that Scott and I have to make big decisions on little information.

The fact that God is using this to draw me closer doesn't make any of those things go away. It does reorient how I deal with this though.

That is what I hope you all see.

Life is hard whether or not you decide to give Jesus the reins. The thing is, He is there and present every step of the way, redeeming every situation, whether we end up seeing why or not.

So anyway, like I said a million words ago, chemo number 2 is now behind us. It went very well. Thank you to those of you who prayed that I wouldn't react.

I had the second round as outpatient, so not only did we not have to stay the night (praise hands), I got to get my chemo in the department I work in.

Seeing my work friends honestly makes it somewhat enjoyable going in to the hospital. It's just one of those detail-things that God shows up in.

Recovery was okay. I didn't wipe out as hard after this one, which is good. Skin pain was still there but not as bad as last time. What was definitely worse was joint/bone pain. I didn't even have to move an inch for my joints to ache.

But today is almost a week out and I've rounded a corner and am on my way to full energy again. My sweet friend Ashley took me to get a shot the day after chemo so Scott could have time to work. She got to see where I work and meet my friends. I love when outside people see what a great place it is.

Tomorrow is wig searching. I don't know that I'll end up wearing one, but the option would be nice. The last place Scott and I went only had old lady wigs. I said "long" and she thought I meant to my chin if that tells you anything. Fingers crossed for good finds tomorrow!

Thanks for hanging in there if you did. I will ask for continued prayers for Scott and I making big decisions. You all are the best.

———

*"Our suffering could possibly save lives. If God's arrow*

*really does go on forever and ever and never ends,*

*it's justifiable that God cares more about*

*our eternity with him than this little pixel today."* [1]

**Jennie Allen**

# RELENTLESS PURSUIT

Jenna was my Young Life leader while I was in high school for all four years, and in that time we grew incredibly close. Looking back, I was probably a rather difficult case, but Jenna was 100% committed to supporting me throughout my faith's journey.

Nevertheless, I was rather inconsistent. I would have periods where I felt like I was on the straight and narrow with my sights set on Jesus and be making so much progress in my walk with Him (all with the help of Jenna's constant encouragement), and then I would wander. I would slip back into my old ways.

My immature, insecure 17-year-old brain told me I was somehow missing out, because pursuing Jesus fully meant I would probably have to give up certain habits and behavior that were hindering.

What I wouldn't give to go back all of those times and reiterate to myself that pursuing some social status over a relationship with Jesus would never make me truly happy, and certainly would not fill the void that only Christ could fill.

But back to Jenna. As I said before, I was probably a frustrating case. Those slipups happened every year. Each time I felt guilty because I knew I had taken so much time and energy from Jenna, only to go several steps backwards. My initial reaction to that feeling of guilt was to be a coward and distance myself from Young Life because I hated the fact that I would have to honestly confront the situation.

But Jenna would never let me. That is not to say she ever forced anything; she just always made a point to reach out and check up on me, whether it was going to a friendly lunch, inviting me over to watch movies, or sitting down and having an honest conversation about the path I was on—which she knew I was better than.

She was so intentional and genuine. She completely took away any fear of judgment I had. She was both a friend and a mentor, and I think it is rare to find someone who can effortlessly be both, and be both so well.

But that was Jenna—a true embodiment of Christ Himself. She was incredibly loyal, loving, and committed when she did not have to be. She welcomed me back with open arms every time I strayed.

She bought me the only Bible I have ever owned and wrote notes inside, reiterating how much I was loved and how joyful and fulfilled I will be if I give myself to Christ.

Jenna is the reason I have a relationship with the Lord, which is the most important thing anyone can have in this life. Her devotion and servant heart saved me from an empty, meaningless life. I cannot thank her enough for that.

*- Ellen L.*

# A video for your Sunday

## 06.28.15

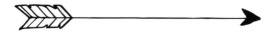

Yesterday Scott and I went to Crossroads with a few friends and the message was given by Steven Manuel. It was really amazing and about the stories we identify with and how we are all called into story and adventure. It is definitely worth going to watch.

That is not what this is about though. On the way out, my friend Ashley reminded me that Steven was the one who gave a sermon on suffering a couple years ago. I immediately remembered because it was one of my favorite sermons. This guy is 2 for 2 on the times I've seen him speak now.

Anyway, I went home and watched the sermon on suffering again this morning, and loved it just as much the second time. I wanted to post a link here so you all could go watch or listen if you had some time today. I hope you do, it's good stuff.

I write this here because I've learned every Word of what he is saying to be true through the trials in my life. If you are someone who wonders about bad things happening to "good" people, or you have been reading along here and wondering how God could let this happen, this is a really good message. Have a wonderful Sunday:)

To watch the video, go to www.crossroads.net and search for "God Is." It is called "God is a Streetfighter." [1]

———

*"The Bible never says if you make all the right choices, life will go well for you"* [2]

**Steven Manuel**

# REVEALED BY SUFFERING

Jenna's battle with cancer provided a visceral picture of the fallen state of our world. This is not the way it is supposed to be, surely this is not what God envisioned when He set to create the world we live in.

Jenna's cancer was not wasted. God did not waste an ounce of her suffering. I am confident that the God of the universe, who is able to redeem and restore all the broken and fallen things, used every bit of her suffering for His glory.

Jenna so beautifully taught me how to walk the line between hope of a different ending and peace with whichever ending God so chooses. While Jenna is often described as our 'sweetest friend,' her gentleness and humble heart was that much more apparent as she walked the hard journey through yet another cancer diagnosis.

Please do not mistake me—Jenna was not weak and she was not naïve. She fiercely clung to her Savior and that is what made all of the difference. She faced the reality of death with hope knowing that her God loved her and was powerful. But she also knew that His ways are higher than our ways and she trusted His heart—His heart toward her. No matter the outcome, it did not change the Truth that her God knew her and loved her. So she fixed her eyes on Him and followed Him to glory.

Jenna did not set out to become such an incredible example to so many, she simply sought to love the Lord her

God with all of her heart. In doing that, she learned how to see the things of this world as fleeting.

Jenna taught me how to hold loosely to the things of this world and to pursue Him with everything. While I do not doubt for a second her love for us, I know that her first love and her true home was not here with us. She knew that even more than any of us and lived out her days eager to be with the one who had her whole heart.

Jenna's battle with cancer taught me that God does not waste our suffering. So often we can be lulled into a state of unawareness concerning the magnitude of the brokenness of our world. Suffering does not allow us the ability to ignore the harsh reality of our fallen world. Watching Jenna's battle with cancer made it impossible to be blind to the fallen state of our world, but it also provides an incredible conduit for the glory of God to be revealed.

Jenna was so faithful. I am not sure I have met someone so consistent with spending time daily with the Lord. I can still see her now, hair piled on top of her head, Young Life sweatpants on, sitting at the kitchen table she painted with her Bible and journal. It was in their daily meetings that God was able to cultivate a humble, but fierce heart in Jenna.

I can remember her sharing during her last months that she could tell such a difference in her heart and day when she did not spend that time with the Lord. It wasn't because it was such a routine part of her day (even though it was), it was because that time with her God was so incredibly sustaining and fulfilling.

*- Randi O.*

# Answered prayers & peaches

## 07.07.15

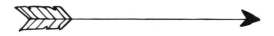

I've been thinking lately about the idea of asking God for big things. It's a scary thing to do, because we don't always get the answer we want. I recently read a book (there have been so many that I can't pinpoint which one. I am going to write a post soon of books that have been so helpful during this crazy time, as well as a playlist that has been great and encouraging) that mentioned one of my favorite passages from the Old Testament.

It's Daniel 3. In it, there are 3 Israelites who refuse to bow down to the statue of the king and worship him. Their punishment for this is to be thrown into the fire. Their response to this punishment was this:

> *"If we are thrown into the blazing furnace, the God whom we serve is able to save us. He will rescue us from your*

*power, Your Majesty. But even if he doesn't, we want to*
*make it clear to you, Your Majesty, that we will never serve*
*your gods or worship the gold statue you have set up."* [1]
### Daniel 3:17, 18 (NLT)

I love their response.

BUT. EVEN. IF. HE. DOES. NOT.

This is the faith I want. Here is the thing: God is good regardless of how He answers my requests. So when I struggle with asking big things of Him, I need to remember that regardless of the outcome, it doesn't change that He is good.

So I'm going to ask for big things. I write this because last night I asked Scott to pray for my hearing test today. One of the chemotherapies I get can cause hearing damage, and since I received this chemo in high school, they are keeping a close eye on it. The one I got before my first cycle of chemo showed that I had some minor hearing loss at a particular pitch. So I asked Scott to pray that it wouldn't be worse.

They told me that ringing in my ears was a bad sign and I've had that ever since my first chemo, so I was nervous. I went to the test today and the guy said,

"You have phenomenal hearing."

The pitch that I couldn't hear before? I could hear it. He triple-checked it to be sure. It took me a few minutes as I was walking out to remember that I asked Scott to pray about that specifically last night. I was pumped.

I went on from my appointment to pick up peaches from our peach guy. Yes, we have a peach guy. He only comes once a year. It's a big deal. Scott was supposed to be the one picking them up, but he ended up not being able to go.

I was kind of sad about going, but I went. The guy that helped me load my car with the boxes asked me if I was in treatment—no hair will do that.

I said yes.

He asked if I was a Christian.

I said yes.

He proceeded to talk to me about how his dad was healed and about claiming the promises in Scripture and it was so encouraging. God literally reworked my day to show up. My hearing appointment was a surprise, we just found out about it less than 24 hours before, and I wasn't supposed to go get peaches, and I did. He is good.

All that to say I am asking big things of the big God I serve. I believe Him big enough to answer, but even if He doesn't, He is still good.

—————

Chemo number 3 starts tomorrow with a 4-day inpatient stay. After this one, we will be halfway done with chemo! There should also be a meeting with the team to discuss and decide radiation, so prayers for those 2 things would be greatly appreciated. Thanks for trekking along on our journey.

*"If we are thrown into the blazing furnace,*
*the God whom we serve is able to save us.*
*He will rescue us from your power, Your Majesty.*
*But even if he doesn't, we want to make it clear to you,*
*Your Majesty, that we will never serve your gods*
*or worship the gold statue you have set up."* [1]

**Daniel 3:17, 18 (NLT)**

# Dear Lord,

## - DIFFICULT DECISIONS -

## 08.04.15

Jesus,

I thank you for the gift that Scott is to me. He makes life a little lighthearted and fun when it isn't and tells me I'm pretty when I feel the opposite.

Thank you for allowing me to walk through life with him. We have this radiation decision coming up. Almost all of me feels like this decision is a no-brainer, but there's a part of me that thinks if you've told me you've healed me, should we or not? Or is that part of your healing?

Please don't leave us in this decision alone. I need you to guide us, Jesus. Show us how to proceed, Lord.

I thank you for chemo being about finished. It's getting harder the further into treatment we get. I cover the last two treatments in prayer, Lord. Smooth the rough places and I pray against any big side effects or reactions.

Please mold Scott and I. Help us not to rush out of this season (as I have been tempted to do). It is in your name I give this, thank you for being good, faithful, and strong, Lord. Amen.

———

*"… He will respond to us as surely as the arrival of dawn*
*or the coming of rains in early spring."* [1]
**Hosea 6:3 (NLT)**

# OVERLY EXCITED

In the summer of 2005, Jenna and I served on summer staff together at a Young Life property in Minnesota. We barely knew each other, but were friends through Lexington Young Life. From the moment that she found out that we were going to be spending the month together, she was over the moon excited. One of those wring-your-hands-jump-up-and-down-in-your-seats type of excitement.

Every time we talked about it together, she would have a big smile plastered on her face with a sense of expectation that couldn't be contained. Now don't get me wrong, I was excited as well, but it's safe to say that I wasn't half as excited as she was.

The day came when we left Lexington and made our way to camp. I'm not kidding when I tell you that Jenna napped on the plane with a grin permanently fixed to her face. Every time she woke up she would comment, "I can't wait!" That excitement didn't fade or die down even once we got to camp. This girl was genuinely thrilled the entire month we were there. There was absolutely nothing you could do to remove this feeling from her being.

She worked the snack shop and loved every bit of it. One night, the shop was opened and Jenna was working. While working, her thumb got slammed in between the screen divider and did a number on her nail bed. It was so bad that she had to go to the emergency room and get stitches. Even as she headed to the ER, she had a smile on her face and was so happy. I'm pretty sure she said, "I love hospitals!"

She returned, gladly ready to talk about it with anyone who was interested and didn't even flinch with the pain she felt. This kind of stuff continued all month long. We bought shirts that matched each other in the camp store and she would plot with excitement which night we would wear them and be "twins." Things like, "I'm so happy!" or "I'm so excited!" were regular phrases heard from her throughout this time and even after.

If I were honest with you, I would have to tell you that for the longest time, I just didn't get it. How in the world could any sane person have this much excitement over the smallest things? Why in the world is she excited to just wear the same dang T-shirt as one of her friends? It's really not that big of a deal! But, as I got to know Jenna and spend time with her, it became evident that Jenna did everything big. She felt all the feelings in a big, big way. She loved all her friends, and served her Young Life girls in that same big way.

Not long after I figured out that this was just who Jenna was: a small girl with a mighty zest and zeal for life, it didn't take me long to want to be just like her. I wanted to find enjoyment, excitement, and joy, even amongst a ride to the emergency room. And if Jenna were here to talk with us about this today, she would tell you that this is all very easy to find if we look to Jesus.

*- Kari C.*

# The middle

08.09.15

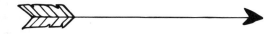

Hey guys. It's been awhile! Thankfully the blog has gotten some use other than updates on how things are going on the cancer front. It has been so good to pick up the camera again. I've been thinking a lot about writing for update purposes recently, but haven't quite pulled the trigger on it. Usually I end up reading something that makes me think, "*Yes! This describes this season!*"

And that is what happened, so I am here to update you.

Chemo number 4 has come and gone, but not without a fight this time. I think the farther we get in, the harder it's been to bounce back. Scott and I went to the clinic to get the shot that keeps my counts from dropping too much the day after chemo (it was the one-day outpatient chemo).

I had been having some random weird symptoms that led to tests we weren't planning on staying for. It is also true that after chemo, when I feel crummy, that my attitude is not the best.

So the day after chemo number 4 was all kinds of a mess. Did I mention that hot flashes are a thing now? Let me tell you, they're kind of awful.

I keep telling Scott I'm done. I'm ready to just be through this and moving on to normal life. Part of me feels like I'm wasting a season of growth by rushing through, but I am not sure that is entirely true. I think sometimes it is ok to just be sad. Most of this past week I have had my energy back and feel like myself again. It's easier to look at the situation from another perspective when I feel like myself.

I'm thankful that the days where I feel crummy and bad are so few. I keep telling myself the more I lean into Jesus, the more He will show up in this process, and I don't want to miss a day of that.

So here we are with 2 rounds of chemo between here and the end. I know that they'll probably be the roughest yet, so I'm enjoying every day I feel great in the meantime.

Radiation should be starting in the next week or 2 if we proceed with that. The weight of what saying yes to radiation means for our family is hitting hard. We have done the simulation for radiation already where they do a CT and make a mold and draw marks on my skin. We only have one more doctor to talk to before we start. Prayers appreciated that Scott and I are listening to the Lord for that decision and not what we think is best.

Here is what I read that made me decide to write. Not everything is exactly how I would describe the situation, certainly not the "beautiful and bright" description of the beginning. But for the most part, I think it's very true that the middle is the hardest, and that's what we're trudging through now.

This is from Shauna Niequist's *Bittersweet*:

> *"There is nothing worse than the middle. At the beginning, you have a little arrogance, loads of buoyancy. The journey, whatever it is, looks beautiful and bright, and you are filled with resolve and silver strength, sure that whatever the future holds, you will face it with optimism and chutzpah.*
>
> *It's like the first day of school, and you're wearing the outfit you laid out last night, backpack full of perfectly sharpened yellow pencils.*
>
> *And the end is beautiful. You are wiser, better, deeper. You know things you didn't previously know, you've shed things you previously clung to. The end is revelation, resolution, a soft place to land.*
>
> *But, oh, the middle. I hate the middle. The middle is the fog, the exhaustion, the loneliness, the daily battle against despair and the nagging fear that tomorrow will be just like today, only you'll be wearier and less able to defend yourself against it.*
>
> *The middle is the lonely place, when you can't find words to say how deeply empty you feel, when you try to connect but you feel like thick glass is separating you from the rest of the world, isolating and deadening everything."* [1]

One thing I will speak to in that last paragraph that has not been true for me is the loneliness part. I feel like God has blessed Scott and I with the best community we could ever ask for. We've had people here every step of the way, and we are so thankful for that.

Thank you, if you have been one of those people for us. I've read a lot of things about people going through treatment and how they say their support disappears after a while. Thanks for sticking around and loving us so well.

One last thing ... at church this weekend they played an old hymn, and the chorus made me cry, it was so wonderful. It says *"Ye fearful saints, fresh courage take; The clouds you so much dread are big with mercy and shall break in blessings, in blessings on your head."* [2] So great.

Thanks for those of you still following our journey. Prayers for no bad side effects or reactions to the rest of the chemo and radiation if we go that route. Also, on top of all the crazy that this past chemo has brought, Scott has a kidney stone, so special prayers for him to pass it soon!

———

*"But, oh, the middle. I hate the middle. The middle is the fog, the exhaustion, the loneliness, the daily battle against despair and the nagging fear that tomorrow will be just like today, only you'll be wearier and less able to defend yourself against it."* [1]

**Shauna Niequist**

# THROUGH FEAR

I had the privilege of meeting Jenna when we were both newlyweds in a new small town, both craving community with other women our ages. Graciously, God provided sweet community in the form of a Bible study with several young women with a heart for Jesus.

Our Bible study group decided to meet at my house during the summer, which put Jenna in contact with our cuddly, but extremely protective dog, Derby. Jenna had a very healthy fear of dogs, but she was brave and came each week to meet, even though Derby met her at the door each morning.

After our discussion that first summer morning, we bowed our heads to pray together. Unfortunately, Derby saw this as an aggressive sign and slowly crept up to Jenna, laid down, and continued a low growl during the entire prayer. We all had our heads bowed, but he singled Jenna out as the most threatening person.

Jenna prayed, but kept one eye open and on Derby the whole time. She was diligent in her prayers, whether she had a growling dog in front of her or not. She saw this as a time she could spend with God, setting her heart to align with His and putting her concerns on Him.

I had the privilege of receiving Jenna's written prayer requests over the next 4 years. Each week, we wrote prayer requests on scraps of paper and passed them to one another to pray over during the coming week. On these sheets, Jenna's heart for Jesus and her love for others shone through, built from the compassion God had cultivated in her heart over years of time at His feet.

She always placed her prayers for Scott, her family, and the teenagers she was loving on first, followed at the end by any requests for herself, even as she was preparing for surgery or working through tiring treatments.

Towards the last year of her life, Jenna's healing was at the top of everyone's prayer requests. Jenna wrote her request for healing in a classic, upbeat Jenna way—with an exclamation point at the end. *Healing!* I still keep the last prayer slip I received from Jenna in my Bible, with the request for *Healing!* at the top. I rejoice each time I see it that Jesus has healed her body whole.

That first summer that Jenna was braving her fear of dogs, we spent our days reading *One Thousand Gifts* by Ann Voskamp at Jenna's request. We practiced writing our blessings and gifts, both big and small. We challenged ourselves to look for the blessings in the hard places of life. Looking back, our hard places at that time weren't fun, but they weren't difficult, compared to what life would bring in the coming years. I am so thankful for that practice during the smooth paths of life, because I can look at Jenna's *Healing!* request and rejoice in all the blessings her journey brought us.

*- Gabe S.*

# Checking in & a few recommendations

## 08.13.15

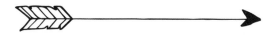

Today is Thursday, but unless I check, I honestly can't tell what day it is lately. Cancer has a way of forcing your life to slow. I fought it for a while, I kept scheming of ways to return to work without ruining my FMLA. After the last chemo, I saw the value in resting and being content with having not much to do.

Today I ate breakfast, read Scripture, had a phone conference with one of our doctors, colored while listening to worship music, and read some blogs. Yep. I do have a photo shoot tonight, so I'll feel a little accomplished later.

Any plans we have usually involve driving to Cincinnati and getting poked for labs, or waiting in doctors' offices. I am ready to get back to normal life, but I am realizing that this time is a gift. Time to rest. Scott's job makes it so he is at home with me most of the time, and that is a gift as well. He's been able to make it to all my appointments with me. This is good because I don't always soak in everything, so a second set of ears is great. I honestly wouldn't be surprised if God gave him the job he has now just for that purpose.

I wanted to take a minute to thank everyone that has sent sweet mail, care packages, gift cards, emails, brought home-cooked meals, driven 2 hours to just hang out and talk. I try to keep up with thank you notes or replies, but I know I haven't been as thorough as I'd like to be. You all have been such a blessing. Hearing from people and having fun mail in the mailbox is huge for me. Scott and I are so thankful for you.

One of our prayers around here these days is that God would provide for us financially. I keep expecting Him to answer that prayer with clients for Scott, but He continues to do so through His people instead. So like Him. I wouldn't be surprised if Scott gets a bunch of clients immediately after treatment ends, so he can be free to go to appointments with me.

If you've sent money or donated to our "GoFundMe" page, we can't say thank you enough. It's interesting being in a place of receiving blessing, rather than being a blessing for others. I hope we've become better receivers through this process.

I've been trying to keep a list of the songs and books that have been helpful for me in this season. These could be helpful to pass along if you know someone who is going through a difficult time, or if you are going through a difficult time and are reading this, you'll have some idea of encouraging things to read or listen to. I know for me, music and books are two of the biggest ways God speaks to me. So today I'll share those, I hope they are helpful.

### Books:

*Every Bitter Thing is Sweet* by Sara Hagerty
*Fight Back with Joy* by Margaret Feinberg
*Bittersweet* by Shauna Niequist
*One Thousand Gifts* by Ann Voskamp
*Walking with God through Pain and Suffering*
by Timothy Keller
*When God Doesn't Fix It* by Laura Story


### Songs:

"Oceans" by Hillsong United
"Shadowfeet" by Brooke Fraser
"How He Loves" by David Crowder Band
"You are Mine" by Enter the Worship Circle
"Desert Song" by Hillsong Live
"O Love That Will Not Let Me Go" by Indelible Grace Music
"Your Hands" by JJ Heller
"Your Love is Strong" by Jon Foreman
"All That I Am" by Rend Collective
"God Moves in a Mysterious Way" by Jeremy Riddle


That's all I have for now. I hope you all have a great end of the week. Prayer requests specific for today are that Scott and I are deciding today whether or not to move my ovary out of the way for radiation. There's a lot going into that decision, so we'd appreciate prayers for discernment for that. Love you all.

*"Go before me and help me to be a good steward of the story you've given me to live out and share."*

**Jenna's Prayer from 6/12/15**

# Dear Lord,

## - MAKE THE ROUGH PLACES SMOOTH -

## 08.16.15

Jesus,

I thank you for a rainy morning, chilly weather, and a front porch. I thank you for your Word and that you are sovereign.

Lord, I trust you. I am sad about the inability to have babies, but I know you have a plan for Scott and me, and I want what you have for us. I pray that we would be content and patient until you reveal what that is to us.

Be working in our hearts and don't allow this to be a bitter root growing in our marriage, Lord. This is in your hands, Jesus. I love you. In your holy and good and powerful name. Amen.

*"We have no reason to complain in any circumstance. God never wastes and He shows up in the most desperate of things to redeem them for His story."*

**A note from Jenna next to Genesis 39:21-23**

*"But the Lord was with Joseph and showed him steadfast love and gave him favor in the sight of the keeper of the prison. And the keeper of the prison put Joseph in charge of all the prisoners who were in the prison. Whatever was done there, he was the one who did it. The keeper of the prison paid no attention to anything that was in Joseph's charge, because the Lord was with him. And whatever he did, the Lord made it succeed."* [1]

**Genesis 39:21-23**

# KIDNAPPED

When I was a freshman in High School, Jenna would regularly pick me and Lauren up after school and take us home. For some reason, we always chose to ride in the back seat together; leaving Jenna alone in the front. For the most part, we behaved.

One day though, we decided to have a little fun. We found markers and wrote "*HELP! We've been kidnapped!*" on some paper and held them up in the window for passing cars to see. I can't even imagine the thoughts of those who drove past our car, seeing two girls holding up these signs.

As the minutes passed, Jenna noticed our giggling and pressed us to share what was so funny. Eventually, she made us show her what we were holding up. Though I'm certain she was inwardly horrified, she laughed and was a good sport about everything. She loved us well, even when we pushed the boundaries.

After this incident, she always made us keep our backpacks in the trunk when we rode with her. No more shenanigans. Jenna was always so patient with us, no matter how much we tested her.

*- Jenna R.*

# Chemo #5 down + radiation started

## 08.24.15

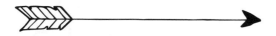

Just stopping in for a quick update. Scott and I got home last night from our LAST INPATIENT CHEMO! So thankful. We officially have one more chemo left. It's not super easy to celebrate yet because today starts the rough week of feeling crummy.

Our last inpatient chemo was spent in a not so fancy room as we've had before, which limited our entertainment options, but forced us to nap more. With the combo of chemo + radiation that is happening now, the threshold for needing blood transfusions is now a hemoglobin of 10, and yesterday mine was 9.6, so I got 2 units of blood. I'm hoping that'll give me a tiny bit of energy to make it through driving to and from Cincinnati every day this week. Well, Scott driving, obviously. The most that I usually do the week after chemo is walk from my bed to my couch, so radiation every day an hour away won't be too fun.

While in the hospital, I had to get transported by ambulance to get radiation on Friday (we went on Thursday before we got admitted), so that was an adventure. It was pretty silly, because it was a gorgeous day outside and would have been a 5-minute walk for us to go, but policy was that I had to go via ambulance.

Radiation literally takes about 3 minutes once you're set on the table. So far no side effects. Other than my hemoglobin dropping so early. The thing I'm going to be asking prayer for is that my counts are high enough to get my last chemo on time. I don't want to push that one back at all.

The nurses on the BMT unit I was on were pretty wonderful. I told all of them to come work in clinic with me. They were very sweet. One night my friends Anne and Shannon were there from Lexington and left at one point after 10:30 pm. Nobody kicked them out. It was pretty great.

Scott and I came home last night to air conditioning that doesn't work, so that is not ideal. At this point I guess we're not surprised. It has been kind of one thing after another since the cars started falling apart awhile back. Hopefully, we can stretch into fall without needing to spend a lot of dollars. Thankfully, this week's weather is going to be gorgeous.

Since we have to drive in for radiation today I am going to start trying to shower and get ready now. Please keep us in your prayers for minimal to no side effects of radiation, especially this week, being combined with post-chemo side effects. I get labs drawn on Thursday, and would like to not come in for blood on Friday, so that's a specific prayer request too.

Thanks friends. Special thanks to our sweet friends who brought us non-hospital food this week. We are so grateful.

*"Blessed be the Lord who has not left you this day without a redeemer ..."* [1]

**Ruth 4:14**

# NEVER STOP ASKING QUESTIONS

The fundamentals of Jenna's life are not things I'm certainly convinced of. I have always struggled with believing Jenna's God was the true God—or even that there is an omnipotent, omnipresent, and omniscient being or even any Creator at all. I hope to make it to assurance; I hope to make it there soon.

However, I can absolutely understand the why behind this season of my life. I've always struggled with not feeling understood, as I have always been a very inquisitive realist who asks too many questions and doesn't know when to quit. Jenna understood people don't "arrive" one day, she knew that improvement is a process.

If this life truly is sanctifying, then it makes sense to have the desire to expand my mind in all ways possible—with close attention to what I hold fast to and what I claim as truth. I truly believe that if God is who Jenna knew God to be, then He loves me through-and-through, without fault, and without pause.

This God is with me here in my disbelief and will not back away from me. My doubt does not scare or worry God, for we both know if the faith is true, I will come to claim it again. Jenna's peace for non-believers makes so much sense to me now. As a Christian and Young Life College leader, I was consistently unnerved by my lack of influence on my non-believing friends and their faith journeys. I had no control and that consistently sent me into fearful prayer. I would prepare, as if cooking a lavish dinner, and then expect my "lost" friends to find that it was just what they had been craving, and be changed forever. I couldn't see God's hand at work in the rebellious and wild lives of my exploring college classmates, nor the goodness that could be bred from making mistakes.

"Never stop asking questions" she wrote in the front of the NIV Bible she gifted to me after my acceptance into the faith at 17 years old, and maybe she didn't know what she was getting herself into, but I have definitely never stopped asking questions. She seemed to love that I inquired about her faith journey, Bible history, and how the world works.

Since I can remember, I have been fierce to figure it out, whatever "it" is. I would question everything under the sun and Jenna didn't back down from my skepticisms; she always encouraged my process. She understood that suppressing one's doubts is not where faith thrives, but rather facing our doubts and being honest about what we think and how we feel can be the greatest good we can do for ourselves.

Jenna has helped instill the confidence to face my doubts and skepticisms in order to better understand objective and universal truths and falsehoods. By this, she has given me a beautiful gift by helping guide and fuel my mental health and depth during critical times in my child and young-adult life.

I celebrate Jenna's life and character as she was an honest leader, a rare heart, and fiercely committed her life and death to divine purposes. As she touched so many lives, there are some she held carefully with both hands and loved hard, all the while crediting no good work to herself.

She met us where we were and loved us enough to share the Gospel, but not without providing a safe space first. She labored, making the dinner plate to set before us, but loved us enough to not force-feed us. I can only hope to imitate Jenna's peaceful nature as I figure "it" out.

*– Ellie S.*

# Final stretch

## 09.02.15

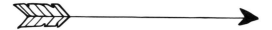

Update time! So, we're approaching the final stretch of treatment, the end is in sight, and Scott and I are going to be SO HAPPY to stop driving to Cincinnati every day. One week from today is my LAST CHEMO and I have 15 more radiation treatments. We are so ready for life to be normal again.

One thing about doing chemo and radiation at the same time is that my counts drop a lot more, since my bone marrow is taking a beating from each. For the first time this whole process, I'm neutropenic this week (*meaning my ANC is below 500, it's 190*).

ANC measures the neutrophils in your white blood cell count. So because of that I've been avoiding crowds and have been wearing a mask when I go to radiation.

Another thing about counts being low is that since the last chemo, I've had to get blood transfusions twice and had to get platelets transfused once. The only fun thing about that is being at work (*I miss it*) and seeing my co-workers.

If you would like to pray, we're asking people to be praying specifically that my ANC would be above 750 next Tuesday and that I wouldn't need platelets. If my ANC is below that, or if I need a platelet transfusion, I can't get my last chemo on time. We really are ready to be done with chemo, so would love it if we didn't have to postpone the last one. Platelets don't last too long after a transfusion, so we're kind of expecting them to be low tomorrow, but hopefully, they'll be on their way up.

In other news, Scott woke up this morning with kidney stone pain again. He still went with me to the hospital, but was having a pretty rough time. He could use some prayer as well.

You can also pray for my attitude as we wrap up treatment. Right now it's great, but I'm dreading the last chemo. After chemo, when I don't feel good, I have been having a pretty awful attitude. Lots of complaining and self-pity and all that. I know anyone would say that I am allowed that, given the circumstances. I do know I'm allowed to be sad, but I don't want to be a person who complains when life isn't easy on me.

I want to be able to take that sadness/whatever I'm feeling straight to Jesus and lean into Him, instead of whining to my husband.

In more exciting news, I have a few things post-treatment that I am looking forward to, other than being a nurse again. I haven't worn scrubs or used any nursing skills since April. I'm ready to go back.

Scott and I are going to North Carolina with his parents and our friends next month. It's going to be the perfect way to celebrate being finished. Then in November, a bunch of my besties are going to Kansas for the weekend. We follow a lady on Instagram who has a craft house and rents it out on weekends. It's basically our dream.

The most exciting thing coming up?? It's basically my adult make-a-wish. *Scott and I are going to the Young Life All Staff Celebration!!!*

When we were told we were able to go, I cried. I'm not kidding. Jen Hatmaker is one of the speakers. Sara Hagerty is leading my seminar. Some of my most favorite people will be there and we get to hang out for a week in Florida. I mean, it is literally the best. Whoever was behind making that happen, know that this is trumping my first make-a-wish of meeting 98° when I was a freshman in high school. So, THANK YOU!

Thanks for sticking with these long updates, friends. We're almost there!

———

"Am I going to let my circumstances determine

my view of God, or am I going to let God

determine how I view my circumstances?" [1]

**Laura Story**

# Dear Lord,

## - AFTER CHEMO -

❧

## 09.09.15

Thank you, Jesus, that chemo is finished. I am so grateful. I know the next few days are going to be rough, so I ask you for your grace and that you'd incline my heart to lean into you, Lord. I pray my stomach would be manageable and not prevent me from doing too much. I pray the radiation would be directly killing every last cancer cell.

I ask for your grace and peace as Scott and I move into a season of remission. Help us to bring any fears, doubts, worries, or anxieties to your feet. Help us to really trust you in this healing you've given. Please forgive any of my unbelief.

Lord, you have been so good to me every step of the way, and I cannot thank you enough for that. Help me to love those around me well, starting with Scott. I pray you'd be working on his heart growing roots and deep trust during this time.

Don't allow either of us to move forward without looking more like you and loving you deeper than we did before. I thank you for the partner you've given me in him.

Lastly, Lord, I ask that you bind the devil from our lives. Command your Angels concerning this household. It is in your holy and loving name I come to you with all I have, Lord. Amen.

———

*"Happiness can be found even in the darkest of times, when one only remembers to turn on the light."* [1]

**J. K. Rowling**

# SCARS THAT HEAL

Jenna was one of my first friends on our unit. She started working about two weeks after myself, and let me tell you, I was a mess with fear, anxiety, and life struggles; I was not sure I would last long on our unit, something just wasn't clicking for me.

Jenna was perceptive to this, no matter how much I doubted myself and my practice. She believed in me. She believed in embracing the flaws and maximizing the strengths of others.

However, my applications were sent out, and I was waiting for a way out, until one day, I accessed a port with Jenna.

We were in a patient's room, about to access a port, when I learned Jenna herself was a cancer survivor.

Accessing a port can be very traumatic and a very vulnerable experience for anyone to endure. This patient, who was a teenage girl, was struggling with the vulnerability and exposure aspect of the port access. As tears were rolling down this patient's face, Jenna held her hand and explained her story; she showed her port scar. She knew, she was part of this "cancer club" that no one wanted to be a member in, she related, she understood.

This moment was a monumental moment for myself. Jenna was practicing on the very unit she was treated on as a teenager, and she came back as a nurse to help others through a terrible situation she endured.

My applications were withdrawn that day.

Jenna wanted to be an oncology nurse, she strived to give the best practice and promote optimal patient outcomes. Through her treatment she continuously had passion for this field and consistently wanted to be back on our unit helping others. Her unwavering faith has inspired us all.

Jenna will always be an inspiration to my practice and it is an honor to have worked alongside her. Jenna, you are a ray of light that will always give me comfort and joy.

*- Kara B.*

# Chemo is finished!

## 09.14.15

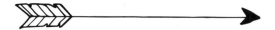

This will be short and sweet. I wanted to drop in to let you all know that I got my last chemo this past Wednesday! My platelets and ANC both shot up way above what we needed them to (thanks for praying!).

Chemo went well, no reaction to either one and it turned out to be a fun day. At Children's, we sing to kiddos on their last day of chemo. Not usually to our adult patients, but because I am an employee, I got the chemo song from my sweet co-workers, doctors, care manager, and social worker.

There were two Cincinnati Reds players that were visiting yesterday as well (with the mascot), so they stopped in to say hi, which was funny in itself, because Scott and I were both older than them. I almost told them I was a Yankee fan, but decided that wouldn't be very nice.

8 more radiation treatments stand between me and the end of treatment, so I'm pumped. I called the FMLA people to make sure I'd be covered through my start back to work date. My short-term disability runs out October 21 and my

first day back is Oct 20. It couldn't have worked out more perfectly.

Today is the 5th day out of chemo, and I'm still pretty wiped out, but hopefully, am starting to round a corner. This time I've had exhaustion, aching joints, and the reflux and metallic taste that have been there for all of them, and then on top of all that, the GI side effects from radiation, so I would say that this has been the worst post-chemo to date. I am thankful that I can stay home and rest though. My only job right now is to recover.

We go to get labs before radiation today, so we're hoping there's no need for transfusions. Tomorrow is our 3-year anniversary, so getting blood or platelets would not be the ideal celebration.

———

*"And he awoke and rebuked the wind and said to the sea, "Peace! Be still!" And the wind ceased, and there was a great calm."* [1]

**Mark 4:39**

# IT DOESN'T HAVE TO STOP

If I could paint a picture of my friendship with Jenna, it would be this. Two girls with long dark hair, driving with the windows down, Chipotle bags at our feet, on our way to the pool. We'd be singing something like the newest John Mayer song at the top of our lungs.

We loved to orchestrate our best days like this. We'd lay at the pool and talk about ministry, and life, and eventually, we both found our husbands, and planned our weddings and futures.

Jenna was my friend that if I wanted to watch the same movie over and over again, she would do it because she actually loved it as much as me. I could always count on her to share with me the best new music coming out, and it would be very normal to hear one of us running down the hall to the other's room, declaring the amazing new song we found.

We sat at our huge kitchen table (that Jenna worked so hard to paint the perfect white) and shared our lives. We served at camps together, went on vacations every year, shared clothes, music, and books. We were in each other's weddings. We did life together for years. I can't think of a single significant memory I had in my twenties that she was not a part of somehow.

She was present and she was so sure. She could also find Jesus anywhere. Looking back, I can see such a steady and mature faith, and I know that was her anchor. She was able to be present and love her friends because she didn't have any doubt about who she was.

With that kind of faith, it's also easy to remind people of the Hope they have and where they are going. C. S. Lewis wrote about this insatiable longing for something that is not on this planet; not in this life. Just as we thirst, we have water. As we hunger, we have food. But we have a desire for this complete, meaningful life that humans have yet to find. Since there is a desire, there must be something to satisfy this desire and because it is not on earth, the inference is that it must be otherworldly.

When you know who you are, who you belong to, and what's ahead, you are able to so freely love others with abandon. I was amazed as I spent time with her the last few days of her life. She exuded peace and joy despite the pain she was feeling both physically and emotionally. I can't help but be changed by that forever.

The beauty of being loved so well by a sister in Christ is that it doesn't have to stop. I can still hear her voice in my life. I still recall moments we had together, and learn from them. I will also never hear a beautiful lyric again and not want to talk to her about it. My joy is that I know she is happy worshiping our Savior now.

*- Holly W.*

# Not quite out of the woods

09.18.15

If you had told me that the worst of treatment would come AFTER my last chemo, I would not have believed you. But that is sadly the truth. The farther I get into radiation the worse my side effects get. At this point radiation has given me temporary colitis, and after making it through 6 cycles of chemotherapy with no nausea or vomiting, radiation has been the thing to make that happen as well.

As of this morning, I only have 4 more radiation treatments left, and I am so very thankful for that. It will take me a couple weeks to recover from the side effects, so it won't be an immediate relief, but I will be on the road to normal here soon. I've been spending lots of time on the couch binge-watching *Gilmore Girls* (thanks Holly). My dreams may or may not include Lorelai and Rory these days.

Scott is attending a conference at our church yesterday and today, and on the way home yesterday his clutch went out. He said it felt like what my clutch has been doing, so we are afraid mine is about to do the same. We kind of started 2015 off with car troubles, and are hoping this is the last bad thing to happen this year. 2015 has sort of been awful for us. That is not to say nothing great has happened, but it has been a very trying year for us.

I am doing the Bible in a year plan from *She Reads Truth* and it has me reading through Isaiah currently (*my favorite*). Today's chapter was so perfect. Well, let's be honest, yesterday's chapter, because I sometimes don't read and then double up. It was Isaiah 40, so right when the book takes a turn for the better.

Half of Isaiah is talking about the unfaithfulness of God's people and judgment, and then you get to 40, and it's God's comfort for His people.

Right out of the gate in verse 2 it says,

*"Speak tenderly to Jerusalem, and proclaim to her that **her hard service has been completed,** that her sin has been paid for, that she has received from the Lord's hand double for all her sins."* [1]

The hard service has been completed part jumped out at me. I know this is talking about Judah's invasion and exile as their punishment, coming to an end, and by no means do I feel like this cancer has been any kind of punishment from God, but the completion of a hard season just resonated with me.

The entire chapter was full of perfect things, and then in closing it says:

*"Do you not know? Have you not heard? The Lord is the everlasting God, the Creator of the ends of the earth. He will not grow tired or weary, and his understanding no one can fathom.*

*He gives strength to the weary and increases the power of the weak. Even youths grow tired and weary, and young men stumble and fall; but those who hope in the Lord will renew their strength. They will soar on wings like eagles; they will run and not grow weary, they will walk and not be faint."* [2]

### Isaiah 40:28-31 (NIV)

If I had to pick 2 descriptors to pinpoint how I feel at the end of this battle, weak and weary would be it. I love all the promises here of renewed strength.

I don't know what is going to happen the rest of this crazy year, but Scott and I are both looking expectantly at God to show up and do a lot of renewing around here.

Thanks for sticking with us, I am excited that the end is so near in sight. Please pray that we'd be able to fix our cars for not an arm and a leg, and for speedy recovery following radiation. Thanks friends!

———

*"Speak tenderly to Jerusalem, and proclaim to her that her hard service has been completed, that her sin has been paid for, that she has received from the Lord's hand double for all her sins."* [1]

### Isaiah 40:2 (NIV)

# Dear Lord,

## - MY LAST RADIATION -

⁕⁕⁕⁕⁕

## 09.23.15

Jesus,

I thank you, Lord, for your Word. I thank you for Isaiah and the way you call your people out from captivity and shower blessings on them.

Lord, I claim those promises for Scott and me as we come out of a season that feels like captivity. Today is my last radiation, and I boldly ask you to kill all cancer cells that may still be lingering. Every last one. I pray for quick healing.

This morning I asked you to give me wisdom and confidence in my interactions, Lord. Give me your words in all situations and boldness in my speaking. I want my life to point to you.

Jesus. I thank you for being good and present in our struggles lately. Go before me and give me grace for the fear that is bound to show up as we move into a stage of remission. I love you, Lord. I thank you that you are a God that sees me. In your holy and powerful name I lift this up to you, Lord. Amen.

———

*"Your face, Lord, I will seek"* [1]

**Psalm 27:8 (NIV)**

# LIFE WELL SHARED

I met Jenna right after she committed her life to Jesus at Young Life camp. From that moment on, Jenna was utterly in love with Jesus. I have honestly never met someone so eager to know the Lord. Given her passion, I felt ill-equipped to lead Jenna in her walk. I remember thinking, "Lord, this girl just met you and already has more knowledge of your Word than I; how can I possibly teach her anything?"

We quickly became inseparable. She became one of my dearest friends; I became part of her family, and she became part of mine. We had sleepovers, shopped for dresses for school dances, talked about her first crush, attempted running (that was a fail, Jenna didn't run!), and went out for chai. There were so many joyful and happy memories, but there were also hard ones.

I remember when Jenna started to feel pain in her side and when she told me that she thought the cancer was back—she just had a feeling. I remember waiting at the hospital, praying it wasn't cancer, though it turned out it was. I knew, though, that cancer would not defeat her. This time, she had Jesus by her side.

I journeyed with her through her second diagnosis of cancer in high school: chemo, sickness, missing school, shaving her head, sleepovers at the hospital. Through it all, she was so brave, strong, and hopeful. After beating cancer for the second time, I knew this girl was going to change the world for Christ.

Although I was no longer Jenna's Young Life leader, we remained close. She was in my wedding; I watched her graduate college; she mourned with me during my son's funeral; she introduced me to this boy she liked a whole lot (of course, it was Scott!), and so many more milestones. Through it all, Jenna blossomed into the most beautiful, gentle, devoted, God-fearing woman I could've imagined. Everything in her life reflected Jesus. She gave her life—to the very last breath—to serve Him.

I'll never forget when Jenna told me her cancer was back yet again. This time, I had a gut feeling that this was it, and I remember thinking that I had to see her one last time. That visit will always remain in my memory. She was sick and feeble and tired; she could hardly walk, and her words were so soft I could barely hear her.

The visit was short—she had little energy, and it was difficult for her to stay awake. In our last conversation, I asked her how she was handling everything: she told me as long as she was in the Word, she was at peace.

As I left her house, I thanked God for allowing Jenna to be part of my life, for showing me what it truly means to be a disciple of Christ—to truly radiate Jesus. The legacy of her life will always be her faithfulness to the Lord, and I know that legacy will live on and continue to change the world for Christ.

- *Kristy R.*

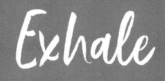

# Exhale

# Finished

## 09.29.15

L̲ast Wednesday was my last radiation! One of my sweet friends texted me that morning congratulating me, and I remember thinking how I hoped I would feel like I was done. When chemo was over, I didn't feel finished (probably because I still had radiation). So, I assumed I may not feel finished.

The whole evening after radiation was finished, I finally felt finished. I think I cried about 3-4 times. Not in a sad way, but in a thankful way. (One of the 4 cries may have been from *Gilmore Girls* though).

The first time I cried, I was feeling really thankful for having literally the most awesome team of people at Children's. I really liked all of these people a lot before they became the ones assigned to me as a patient, but I could not have asked for better people to take care of me through this. All the cries after that were basically the same, me feeling really thankful for the people throughout this process.

My sweet husband basically put his new job on hold for the past five months so that he could be free to go to appointments with me, stay in the hospital with me, drive me to radiation every day, he cleaned our house, did laundry, did all the grocery shopping, all the cooking. He made me feel like not having hair wasn't a big deal. I'm pretty sure he's loved the break of not finding hairs all over the place. I won the husband lottery.

The plan moving forward is scans around 6 weeks out from radiation, and if all looks well, I'll get my port removed after that. I'll keep getting inhaled Pentamidine (really nasty medicine you inhale that helps prevent any infections) for a year because my immune system won't be 100% right away. That is not super fun, but I can probably do it while at work.

I get to be a nurse again next month! I am very excited about that. When I go back, it'll be 6 months to the day from my last shift. That is a LONG break. While I've been on leave we've had some wonderful nurses quit, and that breaks my heart. It won't be the same without them. If you're my co-worker and haven't already left, you're not allowed to leave! No more people are allowed to go!

Healing wise, I'm still on the mend from radiation, and probably will be for another 1-2 weeks. I have good days and bad days. I have tiny eyebrow hairs that look like they're trying to grow back, so that is exciting. I'm hoping hair will start growing back in the next week or so.

So if you've followed along with my story here from the beginning, you've probably noticed that sometimes my posts sound like book reviews. I've read some really wonderful and truth-filled books during this process that have really connected to where I was with everything.

There was a chapter at the end of a book called *Bittersweet* by Shauna Niequist that I loved, about sharing our stories. I decided to write updates and share this story because I've had some friends go through really hard things who have shared them on blogs before, and I've noticed each time that God uses them and uses their story to show who He is when they do that. Kristy, Libby, Kayla, and Holly: thank you so much for sharing your stories and letting God shine through you when life is painful and hard. You all gave me a good example of what God could do if I didn't just keep to myself in this season.

These are the things that stuck out to me from the story sharing chapter of *Bittersweet*:

> "*The big story really is actually being told through our little stories, and by sharing our lives, not just our sermons, we're telling God's story in as reverent and divine ways as it has ever been told. God's story was told in Hebrew and Greek, and I believe that it's also being told in whispers and paintings and blogs and around dinner tables all over the world.*"

> "*My life is not a story about me. And your life's not a story about you. My life is a story about who God is and what he does in a human heart.*"

> "*There's nothing small or inconsequential about our stories. There is, in fact, nothing bigger. And when we tell the truth about our lives—the broken parts, the secret parts, the beautiful parts—then the gospel comes to life, an actual story about redemption, instead of abstraction and theory and things you learn in Sunday school.*"

> "*This is what you do: tell your story. Don't allow the story of God, the sacred, transforming story of what God does in a human heart to become flat and lifeless. If we choose silence, if we allow the gospel to be told only on Sundays, only in*"

*sanctuaries, only by approved and educated professionals,*
*that life-changing story will lose its ability to change lives."[1]*

I hope that if you've been following along, you have seen a bit of who God is through this process. I know that Scott and I would not have been able to walk through this without Him. He truly is a God who meets every need and never leaves us to battle alone.

I don't know how much I'll write from this point out. I am hoping that life gets back to a new normal where cancer isn't something that affects our days in the way it has these past 5 months.

Thank you so much for sticking with us this far, thank you to those of you who've prayed for us throughout this; it truly has made the biggest difference. Thank you for every text, email, comment, card, package, home-cooked meal, check, bouquet, you name it. Scott and I are beyond thankful for every kind word and act of serving us these past 5 months.

If we never got back to you or responded, we apologize, know we are thankful for you. On that note, if you are our family member and did not yet receive a birthday/father's day/mother's day gift, we have not forgotten you!

————

*"My life is not a story about me. And your life's not a story*

*about you. My life is a story about who God is and*

*what he does in a human heart."[1]*

**Shauna Niequist**

# UPSIDE DOWN

I lived in a couple different houses with Jenna in college. Our first house, at $191/mo. each, was horrifically dilapidated. I know that it broke Jenna's sweet mother's heart to come visit us; she was always so sad that it was the best we could afford.

We were just so happy there together, the six of us, that we basically didn't notice. We read books together. We prayed together. We had spontaneous parades. But the house had fleas, it once flooded from the ceiling, the creepy crawlies in the basement were so big that we called them "lobsters," and there were squirrels living in the walls. Once they scratched through into our kitchen, and we duct taped a plastic plate over the hole and moved on.

In our next house, we were ready to move up in the world. People had boyfriends to impress, and we wanted a dishwasher and air conditioning. So we found a sweet little place on a more residential street a little more distant from campus, and from the bars and tattoo parlors that had previously been our neighbors.

I planted flowers out front, and we called it the Hummingbird House—after the street name. Our art student roommate, Emily, moved her nudes (now that's another story for another time) to her own room, and decorated our new place with only her classiest work: a humongous and truly bizarre painting of money, decorated with saints, reading

"THUG LIFE," and a lovely painting with flowers and doodles that, if you looked closely enough, spelled out "sh*#."

Jenna (mostly) quietly tolerated it and decorated the space outside of her room with her own art: the fruit of the spirit (Galatians 5:22-23). I think she was working on memorizing the verses, and I know she was driven to see that fruit in her life. She prayed for it, and she received them. Jenna always surrounded herself, in every way possible, with Scripture.

When I think about Jenna's life, what I think I learned the most about God is the way that God likes to turn things upside down. Many people will tell you that Jenna is the strongest human being they have ever met, and it's true. She approached her school, her career, her friendships, her marriage, her recurrent battles with cancer, and her pursuit of Christ with daring abandon, calm focus, and never one single complaint.

She was a warrior, and I don't think anyone who knew her would disagree. I love that God also lets that person, the person who teaches us what strength looks like, be a small person. A person with a high voice and a goofy laugh. A person whose actual dryer lint was pink. Who put bows everywhere. Who named her pet turtles Molly and Spike. Who was constantly laughing at everything, including herself.

I love that Jenna would not want one single ounce of credit for facing her battles, because her strength came from her relationship with God and her understanding that her life was not about herself.

*- Shannon H.*

# Dear Lord,

## - LEFT WITH SCARS -

※

## October 2015

Jesus,

I thank you for meeting me in the car tonight. I was driving home from Lexington after celebrating Jen with the girls and was thinking about kids (naturally, after seeing all my friends).

I was listening to *"Good Good Father"* [1] and thinking about how I'm going to be dealing with the pain of infertility for a long time and how, even though we're done with treatment, I am left with scars.

But, I thought of child-me when I would play house and daydream about kids and what I would name them and how you knew me even then—before I knew you—and how you knew my story and my heart even in those moments.

I had tears pouring from my eyes and felt in the same moment, so broken and sad about our situation, but <u>SO</u>

loved and known by you. Thank you for that moment, Jesus. I needed it.

You are good, Lord. I pray for a family for Scott and me in your good, good name. Amen.

———

*"From now on let no one cause me trouble,*
*for I bear on my body the marks of Jesus."[2]*
**Galatians 6:17 (NIV)**

# WEEPING HEARTS

Jenna was the sweetest, every time I saw her she always greeted me with a smile and had the incredible gift of making me feel very welcome and comfortable. I loved that about her.

That was a gift of hers, and rooted within her was her hope in our dear Savior. When I think about Jenna, I think about how real that hope really was. Every time I got on social media I would always look forward to reading a post from Jenna. Her words had such truth, and brought so much light amidst such darkness.

Being someone who has been close with tragedy, her words brought me comfort and connection.

Suffering is hard. She did not deny that, but what encouraged me was her constant faithfulness in Jesus' goodness and presence in her life.

*"I love that God weeps and mourns with us.*
*That He walked the path of suffering first*
*so I could look to Him for comfort."*

Such true words written by Jenna. Words that comfort my broken soul, yet lead me to the arms of my God who walks alongside my weeping heart, weeping right along with me.

This is who our God is, and this is who Jenna proclaimed Him to be right until the day she saw Him face to face.

*- Kayla W.*

# Dear Lord,

## - REAL INTIMACY -

01.09.16

Jesus,

Thank you for the gift that is Young Life. I thank you for the ways you are using it to change lives all over the world. I thank you for the challenges this conference is laying on my heart.

I pray I would not walk away unchanged. I pray the same for Scott, that you would speak to him and challenge him where you see good.

Help my heart to fall in love with you as I did as a freshman in high school. I want real intimacy with you, Jesus. Go before me, preparing the way and open my eyes and ears to see you and hear your sweet small voice. Amen.

*And I heard the voice of the Lord saying,*
*"Whom Shall I send, and who will go for us?"*
*Then I said, "Here I am! Send me."*[1]
**Isaiah 6:8**

# REFLECTED LOVE

Jenna was my Young Life leader in Lexington, Kentucky when I was in High School. My involvement in the organization was minimal throughout my time there, yet I would always see Jenna in the lunch room, or the parking lot.

Her constant presence in the school was one of the many reasons I became so curious about YL, so my senior year I began coming around to club and campaigners. Once summertime came, everyone began talking about summer camp and I knew I had to go!

I remember calling Jenna two days before camp asking if it was too late to sign up. Her response was filled with such excitement that it made me feel like the most important person in the world, which was honestly how I felt after every interaction with Jenna.

My life was forever changed after that week spent at a Young Life camp and so much of that is because of Jenna. She went above and beyond for us to experience an unforgettable week, including arranging for the camp mascot to come to our room during cabin time. There we were, 10 high school girls screaming in excitement over a giant whale. We absolutely LOVED it, and that too was all thanks to Jenna.

Jenna was such a beautiful reflection of Jesus, she radiated His love and it was contagious. So contagious that I later became a Young Life leader at a middle school in Lexington.

When Jenna's cancer came back, I experienced a lot of confusion in my relationship with God UNTIL I would see or speak to Jenna. She was steadfast, she was faithful, and she was driven. She battled cancer beautifully. I have never seen anything like it.

After Jenna's celebration of life ceremony, I thought, "*How could someone not believe in our God after witnessing a life like Jenna's.*" The room was filled with so many young women who know Jesus because of Jenna's obedience to Christ, myself included.

Every time I think of Jenna, I smile. She brought so much joy to this world and her legacy continues to do so. I know Jesus better because of Jenna.

- *Meredith B.*

# Dear Lord,

## - AN INTERNAL STRUGGLE -

## 01.13.16

Jesus,

I want to dive deep into this internal struggle with infertility. I don't want to gloss it over and only deal with it when I can no longer keep it down. I've been thinking about Luke 1:45 today. I think I've been taking it to heart to mean you'd give Scott and I a child, whether that be biological or through adoption.

But nowhere in your Word does it say "*Jenna, you will have a child.*" There is a desire in my heart for one, and I lay that at your feet. Jesus, when all is said and done, I know deep in my bones your plan is best for me. So whatever that is, I ask for your great faith to walk in it with you.

On the days where I feel sad, allow me to lean into you. I thank you that you are who you are and not the kind of God I could think up.

Jesus, draw me into your heart through your Word this year. I want to have a heart on fire for you and your Word. I pray it would be the thing I crave. I will show up if you'll meet me there. Do a mighty work in my heart this year, Jesus. In your Son's name, Amen.

———

*"And blessed is she who believed that there would be a fulfillment of what was spoken to her from the Lord."[1]*

**Luke 1:45**

# DESPERATELY SEEKING

Sweet Jenna,

Your life has forever changed mine. To this day, whenever I tell my story I always mention you. How you loved me, prayed for me, and taught me about Jesus. I remember when I first met you. I was 14 and a freshman in high school. I attended Young Life club because my older sister went and it sounded like fun. You were so sweet and welcoming.

At that point, my high school years were just beginning and I was desperately seeking acceptance. I had already begun partying and drinking on the weekends to fit in and feel liked by others. Young Life wasn't like the church groups I had experienced growing up. It was fun and crazy and I got to laugh with my friends, so I continued coming each week. You were always there and would take the time to talk to me and ask me how I was doing.

I went to Young Life camp three times throughout high school, and each time I was in your cabin. The first time I went, I remember being so overwhelmed by the realness I experienced at camp. You would ask us questions about the message we had heard and we would open up about our struggles, from broken home lives to feelings of unworthiness. Tears were shed at every cabin time.

I heard about the hope of the Gospel that week and went home feeling encouraged by the new life Jesus was offering me. You remained constant in my life even though I struggled to follow Him. You invited me to all the Young Life events, continued hanging out with me, and came to my cheer competitions and games.

After my second year at camp, we started a Bible study. I had just spent the week hearing about Jesus and processing the Gospel once again. You helped me read through Scripture and pointed out His promises to me. I am so thankful for those times with you because not only were you teaching me about Jesus through His Word, you were teaching me about Him through your life and the way you loved me so well.

You bought me my own study Bible and wrote in the front cover, "1 Cor. 5:17." The verse reads, "Therefore, if anyone is in Christ, He is a new creation. The old has passed away; behold, the new has come." I had been living an exhausting life of keeping up the image I had made for myself. It was a heavy burden and I wanted to be made new so badly, to ditch this person I had created and be who God created me to be. But I wasn't ready to give up my control.

When I heard the Gospel again at my third year of camp it finally clicked. Because of your investment in my life and God's grace and goodness, I gave my life to Him that week and I have never been the same since.

Now, as a 22-year-old, I have been walking with the Lord and learning from many different women. But your role was special. At the time, I didn't know that as you were teaching me and hanging out with me, you were planting a seed that would grow until I finally realized that hope in Jesus is the only solid foundation in this life.

I can't believe how blessed I am to have learned that from you. You loved Jesus with all your heart. You were faithful and rejoiced in His goodness through all your suffering, even into your last days. You taught me what it looks like to be a woman of God and to trust Him with all that life brings. You taught me that even in the hardest of trials, the Gospel remains true and our joy cannot be taken from us.

Your life impacted mine and countless others. I know that as you entered into heaven, Jesus couldn't wait to greet you to tell you how proud He was of you. I know that with the biggest smile on His face He said, "Well done, good and faithful servant!" Thank you for being there when I needed it most. I can't wait to feast with you at the banquet.

*- Marissa C.*

# Dear Lord,

## - FEAR CAN'T WIN -

02.17.16

Jesus,

I am feeling a lot of things lately. There are moments when I am so thankful that life is good right now, but I feel like I have an undercurrent of fear that I'm living with.

I am afraid of cancer making a fourth appearance, Lord. Even though I know you don't change and will get us through it, regardless of outcome. I know you are good and will be enough. I still don't want it to happen.

I want to grow old with Scott and have (adopt) babies. Those are not ultimate things, you are more worthy than either of those dreams. I guess I need to be living in the moment, being grateful for the blessings you have poured out on me.

Help me to keep my mind from going down a path that is full of speculation and fear. Jesus, go before us tonight. I pray you'd bring kids to Young Life club tonight.

Give me eyes to see where you're moving and boldness to follow. Give me wisdom and discernment. Show me how to best encourage and challenge. I want to be responsible with your Gospel, a faithful servant of your Word and character.

I give you Scott, Lord. Pour blessings down on him. I pray you would be continually drawing him to your heart. I pray for a family. I put all of those details in your hands. You know my heart and you know what is best. I love you, Jesus. In your holy name, Amen.

———

*"Adoration makes walking with God more than just reacting to a series of externals. Adoration calls the circumstances, no matter how high or low, into proper submission in our hearts. Adoration roots us in a reality that no amount of pain and no amount of blessing can shake."* [1]

**Sara Hagerty**

# HER OWN FIERY FURNACE

Jenna has often been described as our "Sweetest Friend." There was always such a gentleness and humility about her. I think sometimes she was underestimated because of her sweet disposition. However, Jenna was not weak and she was not naive. There was a fierceness to her as well.

That resolve became more and more evident as she went into her last battle with cancer. Her gentleness and her fierceness both came from the same source: God. She was faithful to walk closely with Him and He was faithful to equip her with what she needed to face the days ahead of her.

I can remember toward the end of her time on earth, Jenna commenting about how missing her daily time with Jesus would impact her whole day. It was so unsettling for her, that despite how she felt and how little energy she had, she would find a way to get near to Him. She knew that despite us constantly attributing such sweetness and humility to her, it was always the Lord's work in her that we saw. She was dependent on Him and that dependence made room for His character to shine through her.

She was faithful to walk closely beside Him. Not only did that faithfulness help her through each day, but it also shaped her view of the world and her priorities. Jenna clung so tightly to her Savior that while she prayed for deliverance from her cancer, she was at peace with whatever God had planned for her.

She was like Shadrach, Meshach, and Abednego in her own fiery furnace: she knew her God was powerful enough to redeem and restore anything, but she also knew His heart for her was good and she trusted in His infinite wisdom. This allowed her to deem whichever path He had for her as good.

This resolve was not just in the midst of crisis, it was something she committed to and practiced every day. She saw Jesus' example and took it to heart. She eagerly and continually laid her life down for her friends. It was through this selflessness that God's love was continually poured out for others to experience. She did not ever forget the power that the Gospel had in her life and she was eager for others to experience the full life she had been gifted.

The beautiful thing is that it wasn't always in big, extravagant ways. She leaned heavily upon her Savior to direct her heart and her steps. This enabled her to be a faithful friend, a constant source of encouragement and support, pointing us always back to Him.

Jenna did not set out to create such an incredible legacy of faithfulness and devotion, she simply sought to chase hard after God with everything she had. That singular focus allowed her to hold loosely to the world and tightly to Him.

Jenna's fierce love for the Lord motivated her to use all God gave her for His glory—including her cancer. While we were not ready or willing to say goodbye for now to our Sweetest Friend, we rejoice knowing that our deep loss is her incredible gain: she finally gets to meet face to face with her Savior and her Friend.

*- Randi O.*

# 5 months out

## 02.18.16

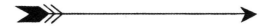

While I've been able to post photos lately, I haven't posted any updates recently and figured 5 months off treatment was as far as I could push it. I think about posting a lot, but have bad follow-through. For Lent I've decided to fast from social media, so that equals more productive time for me, which means updates here. That being said, I'm going to have Scott post an update on social media for me to keep everyone updated.

So, since I've last updated you, I've had 2 rounds of scans (MRI, CT, and PET). Both have come back clear! The labs we drew with my last round of scans came back with an AFP (the lab that we used to call my tumor marker) a tad higher than the last result. Nobody is worried about this, which is great, but I'll be happy to get it redrawn at the beginning of March. I like decreasing trends, not the other way around.

I've been back to work since October and it has been great. I don't think I've ever enjoyed working more. I know it sounds silly having gone through this twice before, but this most recent time has given me a greater perspective at work.

Maybe because the last 2 times I was a teenager and a lot of the applicable memories have faded. I really love taking care of kiddos getting chemo. I have a renewed passion, for sure. I left work today thinking how much I love what I do. I'm even excited about going back tomorrow at 7am. Who am I? That is a huge blessing.

So life post cancer is weird. Those of you who have walked in those shoes absolutely know what I'm talking about. For those of you who haven't, I'll do my best to paint a picture.

In a lot of ways, Scott and I have come out the other end of this thing doing great and bouncing right back. For all the ways that has been true, I am so grateful. I did, however, plan on being able to talk about how we came out with no scars, without even smelling like the fire. I had planned on talking about Shadrach, Meshach, and Abednego from Daniel 3, and how they danced in the fire and came out without a hair on their head singed and their clothes didn't even smell like smoke. I was so sure that was going to be the case, but at this point in time, I don't think I can claim that.

I feel like there are scars left for sure this time. I had not really felt like that before. Scott and I are going to always have to battle sadness on some level about not being able to have kids. 99% of the time I feel at peace about this, but there are times when it is really hard.

One thing I've heard a couple of times these past few months is that motherhood is not my highest calling, Jesus is. That is a truth that I am clinging to. And the thing about it is, Jesus knows my heart more deeply than anyone can. He is the one that has placed a desire to be a mom in my heart in the first place. I don't doubt that He will make that happen in His own way and timing. So I will rest in that, and be grateful for a God who cares so deeply about our lives.

Another thing that I'm not surprised about, maybe just a little sad about, is the anxiety that comes with scans and lab draws post-treatment. I was almost 13 years in remission before, so the scariness of follow-ups and lab draws had disappeared. I feel like we are back to square one, and I forgot what it was like to lose that certainty.

When I have patients now who have follow-up scan appointments, I can understand again that look in their eyes and in their parents' eyes. I get it. We are going to continue to do scans every three months for a while longer. They are letting me draw labs every month if I want to track my AFP. I plan on getting it re-drawn in March, but if it is the same or less, I'm going to stick with every 3 months so I don't drive myself crazy. Prayers are definitely appreciated on that front.

On a happier note, it feels WONDERFUL to be a normal person again. I know I say that a lot, and I don't know if people actually understand how great that statement is. To feel healthy is such a great blessing. There were so many times throughout treatment that I cried because I was just so tired of feeling crummy and tired. Normal is great, beyond great, and I don't want to forget what a blessing normal is.

Another thing I just assume people get, but probably don't, is how weird it is to be in contact with your doctors a couple times a week at least, to "we don't need to see you for 3 months!" Which is a great thing, for sure. And I am so thankful I work with my people every day. It is hard to go from one to the other so suddenly. I don't know why. I don't know if it's because the only real (consistent) contact you have with the outside world for such a long period of time is your healthcare team, or you're used to being monitored so closely and now you don't have a need to be. Who knows. Either way, I'm thankful to work alongside my people, and try really hard not to ask them questions all the time.

It's really weird to think if I get sick now, I can probably just go to my normal doctor, who must be wondering where I've been the past year. So much about cancer makes life really weird.

I'm about done here, but it wouldn't be an update post if I didn't share a book full of awesome truth. I saw my friend Libby recently in Florida (she is 5 years cancer free now!!), and she told me Tim Keller (my fav), had a new book called *Walking with God through Pain and Suffering*. I've only read 3 chapters, but guys. I mean. I maybe have underlined more words than not.

Also, there is a great book by Laura Story called, *When God Doesn't Fix It*. She and her husband have a really amazing story, and such a great perspective.

One last thing. Remember how I heavily quoted a book called *Every Bitter Thing is Sweet* by Sara Hagerty throughout treatment? Well she spoke at the YL conference back in January (which was so amazing and basically my adult make-a-wish), and I got a chance to meet her. I was able to tell her thank you for sharing her story and how much it meant to me during the hard days.

God is good, you all. What a fitting way to start the new year. That's all I have for you. I'll pop back in periodically. Next month there will be WEDDING PICTURES on my blog. I'm photographing my first 2 weddings back to back in March, so get ready for all the pretty things here in a few weeks or so!

Love you all, thank you for reading. I'm leaving you all with a quote from Tim Keller's book. (speaking of the furnace), he writes:

*"Anything with that degree of heat is, of course, a very dangerous and powerful thing. However, if used properly, it does not destroy. Things put into the furnace properly can be shaped, refined, purified, and even beautified.*

*This is a remarkable view of suffering, that if faced and endured with faith, it can in the end only make us better, stronger, and more filled with greatness and joy.*

*Suffering, then, actually can use evil against itself. It can thwart the destructive purposes of evil and bring light and life out of darkness and death …*

*He (Jesus) plunged himself into our furnace so that, when we find ourselves in the fire, we can turn to him and know we will not be consumed but will be made into people great and beautiful."* [1]

———

*"Let your roots grow down into him, and let your lives be built on him. Then your faith will grow strong in the truth you were taught, and you will overflow with thankfulness."* [2]

**Colossians 2:7 (NIV)**

THIRD SEASON

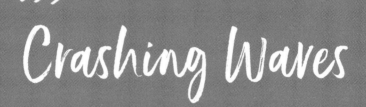

Crashing Waves

# Cancer is the worst

## 03.20.16

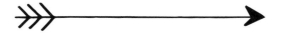

So usually when I sit down to write, I have a direction or theme for my update, and I don't really have that, so bear with me if you're reading the whole thing.

A few weeks ago, I wrote an update about clear scans, but was unhappy about one of the labs coming back slightly elevated. That lab was the tumor marker lab, and we re-drew it 2 weeks ago; it came back even higher. We wanted to make sure it wasn't a lab error, so re-drew it this past week, and it came back even higher.

I had an MRI on Thursday this week, and found out on Friday that I have two 3cm spots that are new. One is adjacent to where the last tumor was, and one is on my adrenal gland.

We hate this a lot. That may be an understatement. When I was in high school I relapsed right after I was finished with treatment, and this feels like the same situation, except that it's relapse number 3.

Thankfully, I work at Children's, so am able to get labs drawn whenever, and am able to talk with the doctors on a regular basis. I keep thinking if I didn't work there, we may have ended up waiting until scans in 3 months, and it would be May before we found out. So that remains to be a huge blessing. And that my doctors are sweet and let me get labs drawn again when I worry.

The plan going forward is not quite made yet. This coming week I will get a PET scan, a CT, and some kind of isotope scan I haven't heard of before. My doctors said the whole solid tumor team has already met and put their heads together about this, which is great. I think they are talking to doctors from a few different places as well.

My tumor is uncharted territory. I think it's something like 0.5% of all ovarian cancers. So, we're asking for prayer for wisdom for the doctors on what to do about treatment.

One thing that has been really great is that the past 2 Saturdays I have shot weddings, so that has kept me really preoccupied. I went into both weddings having just got bad news (increased lab the first one, and the new spots this last one). I have loved keeping my mind off things. I know it doesn't do any good to sit and think about things when they're still up in the air. Pretty wedding pictures have been a very welcome distraction.

Our prayers are for continued peace. We've been angry and sad over here, but have had a lot of peace as well, which can absolutely only come from Christ.

People comment on me having a positive attitude all the time, and that's definitely not it. Philippians 4:7 says:

*"And the peace of God, which transcends all understanding, will guard your hearts and your minds in Christ Jesus."*[1]

Peace that transcends understanding is the only way to describe peace in our situation. We are also asking for prayer for healing. Whether that be instant (we'd love that), or after treatment, we just want healing. Again, wisdom for the doctors. And that God would be lifted high. We'd love if people got a glimpse of who Jesus really is through this. Otherwise, what a waste.

One more thing before I go. When my lab came back increased, my friend Darci called to pray over me via phone, and one of the things she prayed was how this is a huge foothold for Satan in our lives. I agree with that. That same day I was doing questions for my Bible study and it was talking about how it's Satan that sits on the throne here on earth. We see that everywhere we look. On the news, social media, and in sucky things like cancer for a fourth time. But the only thing that matters is that God sits on the throne in heaven. He is the one that will get the last say one day. And that is great news to celebrate.

I'd love for Him to get the last say in this situation like right now, but my timing is different from His. Maybe He will, and that would be great. But I don't even begin to presume what is going on under the surface of all of this, all I know is that He knows, and I truly believe He can take the worst of the worst and show up in that in big ways. He always does.

Also, lets clear one thing up while we're at it. I think a popular belief is that God doesn't give us things we can't handle, and that is crap. I certainly can't handle this. But He can.

And God shows up in mighty ways when we're at our weakest. I've seen it over and over again. He really has been so amazing and faithful in this mess. He's big enough to carry our biggest burdens and strong enough to stand up to our hardest questions.

He is so good. I think you can only know that truly if you've been through what we have and seen Him show up the ways we have. That doesn't mean we can't be angry and sad about this. We are. But He is certainly big enough to handle our angry and sad.

And for that I'm thankful. Thanks for reading and praying. It means the world.

*"And the peace of God, which transcends all understanding, will guard your hearts and your minds in Christ Jesus."[1]*

**Philippians 4:7 (NIV)**

# WORTH IT

*"If only one person comes to know Jesus
because of all this, it's totally worth it."*

This is something Jenna said to me about a month before she died. These words, and the way she lived that out, have impacted my life forever.

I am a different person—a better woman, a better wife, mother, and friend, because of how Jenna loved me. I pray all the time that I too can be all consumed by the Lord. I pray that I can live and love in a way that is bold and unafraid. I pray that my faith is more than just a statement, just as her's was.

What I need you to know is how much Jenna has changed me. I want to be a better follower of Christ because of Jenna. I want to be a better friend. I want to try and find beauty everywhere I look. I want to love my husband better. I want to enjoy all the little moments with my children. I want to be brave and bold and have the faith to step out and have hard conversations with people. I want to ... and I have been.

God has used Jenna to change our lives. I will never forget all the people who stood at her service because they knew Jesus better because of her. It took my breath away.

She affected generations. My kids pray for you, Scott, and talk about her all the time. Her memory lives on and will continue to live on through all those people who stood and all the people who are continuing to be impacted by her story.

I miss her. But I also can't help but smile thinking of her now and the joy she has, the pain she is without, the worship— just every way she's experiencing life with Christ right now.

Thank you for sharing your lives with us. Thank you for sharing Jenna.

*– Darci M.*

# The rough plan

## 03.27.16

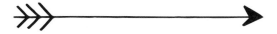

So we've learned a whole lot since I last left you with an update. We met with my team on Thursday night this past week. This past week consisted of a PET scan, CT, Octreotide scan, labs, and then sitting down with my doctors and care manager to talk about all of the above, and what we do moving forward.

No surprises on the PET scan. Just the 2 spots we already knew about that lit up. The CT of chest was clear. The Octreotide scan had one of the spots lighting up (I'll explain further in).

First things first, my doctors are a huge blessing. They've been tirelessly working, reaching out to doctors all over the country (and in Germany) to get opinions from the best of the best. These doctors have been so generous in sharing their expertise and being willing to help. I could not be more thankful for that.

Without getting too detailed, there are 2 opinions about what my cancer actually is. The doctors at Children's all agree it's a Sertoli-Leydig cell tumor, and that is what we've always known. It does have some atypical features that look like a neuro-endocrine carcinoma. The good news is, the treatments for each kind are very similar. So either way you look at it, we'd be approaching treatment the same way. (The one spot that lit up on the Octreotide scan would point to neuro-endocrine carcinoma).

So to start, surgery is this coming Friday to remove the spots and look around to see if there is anything else the scans didn't pick up. My surgeon ran down to clinic while I was working this past Friday to answer a few questions and touch base before surgery. He is hoping to do this laparoscopically, which would be a much quicker recovery, but will have to do open if there are areas he needs to get a closer look at. So my inpatient stay after surgery will be anywhere between 2-7 days, depending on what ends up happening.

I don't even want to start about the new visiting policy. Scott may throw a fit and embarrass me. You can only have 6 people total on your list of visitors and how in the world are we supposed to work with that? Yikes.

After surgery, the rough plan for chemo involves 2 oral chemotherapies and one IV chemo. The side effects of these are not as bad as the ones I've received in the past, and I will hopefully be able to keep working and being a normal person during treatment. Hair loss is not a huge side effect for any of them, so we're hoping that won't happen. The plan is that if I'm tolerating them well, we would do these for 2 years.

I don't like that, but if it's not as bad as the ones I've had in the past, I think that could be doable. The doctors believe this is something that will keep coming back, and that we'll continue to fight it.

We are praying for healing over here though, and hoping that is not the case. In John Piper's *Don't Waste Your Cancer*, he says, "you will waste your cancer if you seek comfort from your odds rather than from God."[1]

You all have already been blowing us away with sweet words and actions. I received 2 adult coloring books on Thursday, each with Scriptures of God's promises. I mean, does it get better than that? One came with a beautiful scarf that was ordered from one of my friends who runs an Etsy shop. So not only did I get a pretty scarf, it supported my sweet friend Cory's business (find her on Etsy, Eclectic Joy). Win-win (thanks Susan). We've received letters with gift cards (mail is my favorite). You all are seriously the best.

One thing everyone should know about (maybe just girls), is a podcast I found by being on Jen Hatmaker's email list. It's called "The Happy Hour" with Jamie Ivey. Jamie interviews a bunch of women, and just talks about life, their stories, what they're loving, what they're learning. It's magical. I love listening on my commute to work, I feel like I'm having a conversation with my friends. I've listened to all of the ones where she interviews Jen Hatmaker, because, of course.

But one other one I've listened to is where she interviews Jami Nato. I follow Jami on social media, and her story is incredible. It's not about cancer, but the truths she's learned through her own pain are so great, and I loved listening to her share it. Two quotes from her happy hour …

*"The only way as a human you can be really close to God aside from some supernatural gift He gives you in a moment here and there is deep, deep suffering. I really believe that, it's the only way you know how near He is."*

*"When things get difficult, really difficult, don't look inward. Don't believe in yourself, wake up and try harder, the answer is not inside of you but outside of you. Simply ask God to show up and change your heart and mind."* [2]

Such good things. Lastly, Happy Easter! Easter has long been my favorite holiday. Scott and I went to Crossroads for their Easter experience last night and it was so great. A little while ago our church sent a team over to Jerusalem and took footage in all of the areas that Jesus lived and died and rose again. It was just really amazing seeing it with my own eyes.

What a great reminder it is of what He has done for us. It brings such great perspective. I can easily look at our situation and say it isn't fair, but the thing that really isn't fair is that Jesus traded places with me and took all of the punishment I deserved so I can get all the life and closeness with God that He deserved.

What can I ever complain about in light of that? He has never owed me anything, yet has given me so much more than I deserve already. Living in the times we do, entitlement is a real thing, and I need to fight that mindset with the truth of the Gospel daily.

Thanks for reading. We are asking for prayer for healing, for continued wisdom for all the doctors involved (mine and the ones on our case in the US and Germany). For continued peace, for the adrenal tumor to be in the peritoneal cavity and not the retroperitoneum. For a quick surgical recovery, for my surgeon to have eyes to see what he needs to see when he goes in. Your prayers mean so much to us. We love you all.

---

*"When things get difficult, really difficult, don't look inward.*

*Don't believe in yourself, wake up and try harder,*

*the answer is not inside of you but outside of you.*

*Simply ask God to show up and change your heart and mind."* [2]

**Jami Nato**

# Dear Lord,

## - PRAYERS ON EASTER -

## 03.27.16

Jesus,

I praise you that you did not stay dead. I praise you for conquering death for me. I thank you for Easter and the great reminder it is of the Gospel.

I am sorry for all the ways I live entitled when you've already given me way more than I deserve. Use me for your glory, Jesus. I want people to know you. Help Scott and I to be lights in every dark place we encounter.

I specifically ask you to reveal yourself to those on my team and in my workplace that do not know you. I lift up all of our Doctors, give them wisdom, and I pray you'd show them your character and power through working a miracle of healing in me.

Go before me this week. Help me to soak in your presence and soak in my last few days moving around freely and easily for a bit. I give this all to you, Lord. Stay close. In your Son's amazing and holy name. Amen.

———

*Jesus told her, "I am the resurrection and the life. Anyone who believes in me will live, even after dying. Everyone who lives in me and believes in me will never ever die."* [1]

**John 11:25, 26 (NLT)**

# FROM ONE TO ANOTHER

I met Jenna in 2006 when I moved to Lexington, Kentucky to live closer to my boyfriend (now husband). She, along with all the female Young Life leaders, welcomed me right into the fold of their community. I am so grateful for that season of life and what I learned about fellowship with women and true community.

When I think of Jenna, I have two distinct memories. Our time in the same place was only 11 months long, but because of Young Life, we saw each other throughout the years. In 2010, I was diagnosed with cancer and sweet Jenna sent me shampoo. It was shampoo to help hair growth after I lost most of my hair during chemo. It was so appropriate for one cancer fighter to another ... to share in the pain and sympathy of hair loss. She read our blog, prayed, and loved our family through one of the most trying seasons of our life.

In 2014, my husband and I were at the Young Life camp, Timberwolf Lake, in Northern Michigan. Jenna was there with her Young Life girls and all week she was glowing, smiling, and loving people around her. Her heart for people and the Lord was the most evident thing about her life. I hope to love others with the intentionality she showed.

– *Libby R.*

# Dear Lord,

## - BEFORE SURGERY -

04.01.16

Jesus,

I thank you so much for the ways you showed up last night through the community you've given us. I thank you for a home-cooked meal and for everyone coming to pray.

I boldly ask you to move mountains today. I pray for healing and I pray for your glory to be seen. Be the doctor's eyes and hands today, Lord. I pray he can do what needs to be done laparoscopically. I pray there are no other questionable spots. I pray for no NG tube, no pneumothorax (collapsed lung).

Go before us today, prepare the way. I thank you for the way you come close in pain. Be close to us this coming week, Jesus. Make your name be known. Help Scott and I to be a light to everyone we encounter. I love you, Jesus. It is in your good and powerful name I give myself to you this morning. Amen.

———

*"The Lord your God is in your midst, a mighty one who will save; he will rejoice over you with gladness; he will quiet you by his love; he will exult over you with loud singing."* [1]

**Zephaniah 3:17**

# DISTANCE RUNNER

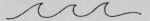

I love to run ... most days. In the moment, I love the feeling of accomplishment, the release of stress, and the time of solitude. But some days, it is hard. I'm in pain, I feel tired, I am discouraged, and I don't have the motivation.

Following Jesus can be the same way.

I love to follow Him ... most days. I love knowing the eternal benefits the relationship brings. In the moment, I love the feeling of peace, the freedom it brings.

But some days, it is hard. I am in pain, I feel tired, I am discouraged, and I don't have the motivation.

Jenna often comes into my heart and mind when I am running. I hear the worship songs she loved, and I think of her sweetness and strength ... her supply of endurance, lack of complaining, focus on Jesus, and love for others.

Thirteen years ago, Jenna bounced (maybe literally) into Young Life Lexington with that beautiful smile and endearing personality. She had a deep love and understanding of Jesus most other eighteen-year-olds don't have or even care to have. Learning about her battles already fought against cancer in her short life gave context to that faith.

I had been leading a Bible study of Young Life leaders for about three years by the time Jenna joined our group. As a Bible study leader, there is an unspoken expectation that you disciple those you are leading. You run in your faith at a pace a little out in front of them, and as you follow God and run at your pace, they follow behind you.

You meet at Panera and talk about the importance of quiet times, the difficulties with roommates, the struggles of changing majors, the journeys toward dream jobs, and the longing for husbands. You offer guidance, encouragement, prayers, and "wisdom." They grab ahold of your faith, in a sense, and let you lead them along until pretty soon they are running beside you. And then you are running together.

You get to read at their weddings, hold their babies, and watch them live out their faith in life. You study Scripture together, and you learn from their growth. You stop calling yourself a Bible study leader, and you start calling yourself a Bible study facilitator.

I loved running beside Jenna. She loved to extravagantly give of herself to her friends, her family, her co-workers, her patients, and her Young Life girls. And that never slowed down for a minute when she was sick.

She poured out prayers for others, wrote letters of encouragement, spoke words of life, and cared for others at every stage of her journey. She went to Young Life camp when it seemed impossible ... because she loved one girl SO much.

So what do you do when your "disciple" starts to outpace you? When her faith seems to run deeper than yours? When her trust in the Lord does not waver when your own seems shaky? When her words of confidence in God's goodness drown out your questions of His plan?

You follow her.

You grab ahold of her faith and let her pull you along as she sprints through the finish line. And you realize that "leader" was never a good title for the role you got to play in her life.

You follow behind her graceful strides as she crosses from temporary to eternal, and you sit in awe and wonder at the impact of her legacy. And as you move forward in grief and loss, you try to imitate the rhythm of those worshipful strides.

So now, I am running behind Jenna as I follow after Christ. I am trying to honor her legacy and seek after Him with the same sort of purity and vengeance that she displayed.

To be honest, it is really hard to keep up with her pace. But she has shown me—in her life and in her death—that without a doubt, all of the running is worth it.

*- Mandy S.*

# Post-surgery update

## 04.04.16

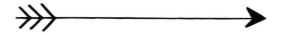

Hello, world! Just checking in from the hospital. Surgery went great. The one mass was not in the retroperitoneum, and not even on the adrenal gland, so it was simple to take out, and the other one came out easily as well. AND I got a bonus appendectomy. Deal.

Recovery has been great. I've been up out of bed since Saturday. The sites aren't hurting, the only pain I'm in is from the port. I asked for it to be on my rib cage (so maybe I can access it myself), and I think that is just a tender area stretched a bit too far. It should get better with time.

Scott and I have had some sweet visitors and all kinds of treats, which I'm just now able to eat. We are really hoping to get sent home tonight, we'll see what happens.

Not much else to report. Thanks for sticking with us over here. We appreciate your prayers, really the surgery went as best as could be expected and recovery is already seeming quick. We appreciate your prayers so much. I'll write more later, but wanted to pop in to say hello.

•

*"I am [in your world].' said Aslan. 'But there I have another name. You must learn to know me by that name. This was the very reason why you were brought to Narnia, that by knowing me here for a little, you may know me better there."* [1]

*C. S. Lewis*

# Dear Lord,

## - RAGING STORM -

## 04.29.16

Jesus,

I thank you for the reminder that when you approached the disciples in the storm, you did not calm the waves but instead invited Peter to step out onto the waves.

We are certainly in a storm with no calm in sight right now, so my prayer is to set my eyes on you so I can stay on top of the stormy waves. Be my peace and calm in the chaos. Amen.

---

*"Because he bends down to listen,*
*I will pray as long as I have breath!"* [1]
**Psalm 116:2 (NLT)**

# CAR RIDES

One early September morning in 2016 I quickly threw some items into an overnight bag and drove to work. I got to the office, pretended to check my email and looked at my phone about every five seconds. I was waiting for the "go" from Jenna's Entourage to hop in my car and drive to Cincinnati.

The previous weekend, Jenna was admitted into the hospital, and we all waited to hear if there was a time when we could visit her.

Around 10:30 am, the imessage banner flashed across my screen and I frantically gathered my things, hopped in my car, and hit the road.

I met Jenna our freshmen year of college and we were both going through first-year training for Young Life. The first time we met, Jenna picked me up from my dorm and drove me to training. When I looked over from the passenger side seat, she smiled and in her semi-silent voice with a little shrug of her shoulders, said "Hi, I'm Jenna," with a big grin on her face.

Jenna had her hair pulled back in a ponytail and two sponge curlers on each side to curl her bangs ... I thought "Who is this girl?" I quickly learned that Jenna is one of the most humble, loving, compassionate, and strongest women I have ever met.

Every Sunday for five months, she graciously drove out of her way to pick me up—to the point where I felt I was becoming a burden to her. We talked about her love for Jesus, Billy Joel, and the Yankees. We bonded over our love for Chipotle—fun fact: Jenna went to Chipotle so much our freshman year that they 1) knew her order and 2) gave her the employee discount—even though she wasn't an employee.

In the middle of our first semester, I started to get homesick. I was six hours from home and trying to figure out where I fit in-college. I felt like I was making friends with people in my dorm but not really connecting with other people in our Young Life training group. On Thursday afternoon, I called and gave some lame excuse on how I couldn't go that week. Jenna listened and said, "I understand."

And in true Young Life fashion, she showed up on Sunday, like clock-work, and said "I am outside and not leaving without you." Jenna, in her meek and humble ways, is one of the most persistent people I have met.

The thing Jenna is most persistent about is making sure people feel and know the love of Jesus. Without Jenna's persistence towards me and our friendship, I would have never been a Young Life Leader or started WyldLife at a nearby middle school. I would not have the friendships I have with the Lexington girls I have today—a friendship that is often indescribable, the way a group of women truly love and live life together.

When I finally made it to the hospital that September day in 2016, I met Scott in the lobby with a few other girls. He looked at me and said, "Jenna told me you weren't coming because you live in Chicago. It's too far."

I chuckled and thought, 'Well, Jenna is in for a bit of a surprise.' When I walked into her hospital room, her eyes opened wide as she said, *"Sarah! You're from Chicago ... how did you get here!?!"*

I simply responded, "I drove to see you." Jenna smiled and said, *"That's far,"* and I told her, *"Well, you're worth it."*

I then sat next to her hospital bed and for the first time told Jenna the story I just shared above. How, without her, I would have not been a Young Life leader—a mission that is dear to both of our hearts—or have the lifelong friendships that I have today.

During the last few days of Jenna's time here on Earth, an A. W. Tozer quote was in a devotional I was sent, it read *"What comes into our minds when we think about God is the most important thing about us."*

Over the past year, when I reflect on what God has been teaching me, Jenna's faith and the way she lived continues to come up. She is still teaching me so much about fearless love, faithfulness, and how to find joy in suffering.

*– Sarah S.*

# Chemo update + turning 30

## 05.02.16

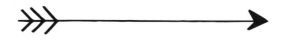

Hello! It has been awhile since I've updated. Oral chemotherapy is underway. I am on day 12 of 14, and am so ready for the 14-day break. It has not been bad, so I can't complain, it's just a lot of staying on top of when to take them, one of them you have to take with food, and one on an empty stomach, and you can only take Zofran (anti-nausea medicine) so often, so I've been trying to be super organized about it.

We've been in the ED at Cincinnati Children's Hospital a little more than we'd have liked a couple weeks back for dumb shoulder pain. It was nothing, so we shook it off and moved on with life, just really annoying having to drive to go and then sit and wait.

This past weekend I turned 30. I feel kind of sad about that because I used to think 30 was ancient. But turns out I still feel the same. Our friends and I always joke that we feel

22, but then we're around 22-year-olds and realize maybe we don't.

My sweet friends came to Indiana to hang out with me for my birthday. They came from Lexington, Louisville, and Colorado (Randi was in town for a wedding!). They walked in the door and started decorating my house with gold (golden birthday). They cooked, cleaned, brought me sweet gifts; we ate Thai, gave Julie's sweet daughter her first dot cake, which was a hit. We had a slumber party and talked in my room until almost one in the morning (which Scott loved ... can you hear the sarcasm? Poor thing just wanted to sleep, to which my friends kept saying, *"There are so many places in this house for you to sleep!"* as they sat on our bed. hilarious).

I joined some sweet co-workers for painting on Sunday; it was so fun. We made beautiful creations. Then I came home and our Bible study met and had a little grill out (with more dot cake). It was so great.

Scott and I went to this year's Brave experience last week. It's a thing our church put together where you go and put on headphones and follow prompts that go with the different rooms you walk through. It's pretty amazing to just slow down and have that time with God. The thing that struck me most from that correlated with the sermon from a couple weeks prior. When Peter walked on the water toward Jesus, the disciples were all in a boat in the middle of the storm when Jesus showed up. What they wanted was calm, and they knew Jesus could calm the waters, but that is not what He did. I relate.

We'd love some calm waters over here. But instead of making life easy and comfortable for them, Jesus called Peter out on the raging waves with him. I feel like that is what He is doing with us. Not calming the waters for sure, but He's not leaving us anxious and worrying.

He's calling us to Him on the waves, where its super scary, but where life is offered. A closeness to Him. One of the prompts said, *"What does He have for you in the next step?"* I love that. Not "How fast and painlessly can you get through the next step?" So we are over here praying that we will be looking for what He has for us, no matter how crazy it gets.

He never wastes trials. Every crazy and bad thing that happens in Scripture is always pointed back to His glory and goodness. This is no different.

———

*"And Peter answered him, "Lord, if it is you, command me to come to you on the water." He said, "Come." So Peter got out of the boat and walked on the water and came to Jesus.*[1]

**Matthew 14:28, 29**

# Dear Lord,

## - IT'S DIFFERENT THIS TIME -

## 05.04.16

Abba,

Today was hard. The cancer is back in sheets lining my peritoneum and they cannot surgically remove it. It's aggressively growing.

Our chemo plan was not working. It is resistant to chemo. There are no cure options on the table. These things are awful.

BUT, you are good, and you are mighty. And zero odds are exactly where you can show up in all of your glory. I praise you for the team at Crossroads that prayed over us today. I thank you that you heard our petitions of healing.

I thank you that you are more than able to heal me. I boldly ask that you did, and will. I thank you for telling us you are pleased with us, I thank you for the affirmation of being a cord of three strands with you. I thank you for the vision of the boat heading towards the harbor away from the storm. I pray we'd keep our eyes on you and not turn back to look at the storm.

I thank you that my name means "God is gracious." I pray that would be a banner over my life. I pray people see that in me and in my story. I praise you that you delight in me.

Jesus, we are at the end of our rope here. I can't rely on experience. I can't look forward to a cure date. I can only lean into you. I thank you that you have not left us alone, I thank you that you are in this with us every step. I give myself to you, Jesus. Heal me. Make yourself known. Be my rock every second, for I am wholly dependent on you.

Your daughter & beloved
- Jenna

———

*"Joy means holding on to hope in God regardless of the outcome. Declaring we will give up everything and entrust ourselves more fully and wholly to the One who holds all things together."* [1]

**Margaret Feinberg**

# IT'S ONLY TEMPORARY

Sometimes when people are gone we tend to rewrite history a little, making them out to be more than they were, or only recalling the best qualities of their life. Not to say that Jenna didn't have a single fault, but what's written in this book isn't a sugar-coated, rose-colored remembrance of our friend. These pieces are her real, authentic self, all the time.

She had the purest heart. It was all I'd ever seen from her, starting when I met her in 2004 as we entered college as tiny baby freshmen, all the way through the week in 2016 when we could see the end was near.

Even in the midst of being sick she'd ask about others first. She always lifted everyone up, encouraged them, encouraged me. She had every believer she knew praying that her medical team, family, and friends, who hadn't yet clung to Jesus as their Lord would see her life and see Jesus for who He is. That they would come to understand the good news, the Gospel of grace, by seeing how good her Jesus was, even in hardship.

At a time when you could become so inwardly focused and downtrodden, she had the ability to see the big picture with clarity. She suffered in such a way that made people ask *why*?

Enduring the pain of cancer, the uncertainty ahead with her health/life, the side effects that come with treatment, the "unfair" hand of four rounds with this terrible disease—why did she have hope? Why did her faith only grow stronger?

Jenna understood the reality of heaven. She believed God's Word with every bit of her being that heaven is not a lesser reality than what we have here, but a far, far greater one. THIS life here is temporary, this is the vapor, this is the shadow, the dim reflection in a mirror. For Jenna, what was to come wasn't terrible.

Of course, she grieved for the people she'd be leaving behind and the dreams she envisioned for herself, but for Jenna this "end" wasn't an end. Leaving this "tent" meant coming face to face with everything she lived for since she was a teenager.

She knew heaven is abundant life without the trappings of sickness and sin. She knew she'd be feasting and running with a renewed body. Most of all, she knew she'd be communing with her Savior, her Lord, her King forever; everything she was made for. Everything each of us was made for.

My favorite part of Jenna's celebration of life service was when our friend Marshall said, *"Jenna would want you to know that she's not in heaven because she was a good person. She is there because she believed in Jesus and He kept his promises to her."* This is so true. She would want you to know that.

The world is less beautiful, less kind, less optimistic without Jenna, but the impact she had in her 30 years of life will ripple throughout eternity, multiplying more grace, more humility, and more hope. I can say with assurance that when Jenna knelt before the King of Glory, He looked at his lovely and precious daughter and said, "Well done, my good and faithful servant."

*– Jen B.*

# Worst news

## 05.05.16

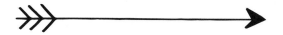

I have absolutely no idea how or where to start this. Scott and I got as bad of news as you can get. We had labs and scans this past week. The tumor marker lab was up to 33 and the MRI showed more evidence of cancer. Not in its usual form of small masses, but in sheets lining the peritoneum and that had traveled up past the diaphragm by my lung.

In this form, surgery is not an option. We are also looking at a 2-week separation from when the tumor marker was 8, so it's a very aggressive and fast-growing cancer.

We found this out on the last day of oral chemotherapy, and so because of that, we knew that those drugs were not working, and because of my past history and the way this tumor keeps evolving, we know that no chemotherapy is probably going to touch it. We also know that radiation did not touch it. So surgery, chemo, and radiation being off the table, we are left with clinical trials and targeted immune therapies.

All of this is really hard to swallow, but one thing I love, and I mean this, is that when all of our options are essentially off the table, it sets the perfect stage for God to do His thing. (Can I just say real quick that multiple friends texted me without knowing when this was going down, saying God had me heavy on their hearts?)

As of yesterday, the plan was to get me into a clinical trial in Columbus. My doctors called this morning and said that I don't qualify for those, but then presented me with alternate plans, and what we're going to do is essentially do the same thing that the trial would do, but at Children's and starting tomorrow. The only difference is the drug I will get is a cousin of the one the trial is testing. And that combined with the IV "chemo" that I was planning on getting before all of this.

The thing we really love is that a trial would necessitate a 3-week treatment break, and this way we can start now. With how fast this thing is growing, I am all about that. And I get to stay at Children's. So we are all on board with this.

With all of these things, the goal is to slow growth and shrink the cancerous areas. There is still a lot of research going on behind the scenes, that hopefully we will learn things from along the way. A tiny mouse somewhere has my tumor and is getting lots of drugs thrown at it to see how it responds. Which sounds sad, but I think is kind of cool (sorry to all my animal loving friends).

A doctor in Michigan wants me to take a supplement that is being studied for use in these tumors, when I looked up what it was, turns out frankincense is derived from it, and I am all about the essential oils, so I'm ok with that. You can get it at GNC so that's also great. I would be the first human test subject, but as it's a supplement people take anyway, why the heck not?

So back up to yesterday, it was a really hard day. Lots of tears is an understatement. I didn't even walk around visiting friends in clinic, I actually hid in my room, even asking my doctor for a warm blanket instead of venturing out to get one myself. Man, we love our team there. We are so blessed by them.

We left the hospital and headed to our church, which thankfully is only 15 minutes from the hospital. We had a group pray over us, and it was so great. I mean like I used 8,000 tissues, but great.

A few things stand out about that. One of the men on the prayer team said he got a vision while we were praying (my favorite when that happens). He said he saw Scott and I on a boat out at sea and we were heading toward the harbor, outrunning a storm behind us. He said that God told him we need to keep our eyes on the harbor, because looking back at the storm leads to danger of hitting rocks on the way in. I love that because it's saying we need to lock our eyes on Jesus, because He is our safety. It does not help drowning in the sadness and craziness that is this storm.

A few people shared some verses that were super encouraging, and at one point, one of them even looked up the Hebrew meaning of my name. Jenna in Hebrew means "God is gracious." I mean, come on. That couldn't be any more perfect. Mom and Dad, you thought I was Jenna because you liked the name. God was thinking other things. They talked about how my life was a banner flying for how gracious our God is. Just. I can't even.

Scott and I read through the story of the bleeding woman and dying daughter in all 3 accounts in the gospels last night (given to us to read by the Crossroads prayer team). Two people with stories we can deeply relate to, and Jesus right in the middle of both of their stories doing His thing, even when it didn't make sense to the man who wanted to rush home to his daughter.

This morning I opened to Isaiah, which I've been reading through. And by reading through, I haven't read it in like a month, but I had stopped at chapter 38, so when I picked up there today it was clear that God used my procrastination for sure.

King Hezekiah was pleading and weeping with God after hearing a death sentence, and 38 flows into 40, which is filled with God's comfort for His people. Perfect.

So in all of our experience with cancer, we've leaned heavily on God for sure, but we also were on familiar ground, where there is a certain amount of floating through easily involved. Not to say we floated through easily, but hopefully you get what I'm saying. This time Jesus is literally our only lifeline. It is a scary place to be, but also what a freaking blessing?

We are still really heartbroken over here, but have peace today. Only Jesus can bring peace in these situations. My peace doesn't rest in treatment plans, but in the God who put skin on and suffered so that He can live with me and in me and fight for me. He is good.

Healing or not, He is good. If you would pray with us, we are praying for the miraculous that only He can do, the healing only He can give at this point. And whoever is praying peace over us, keep it up. It's working.

———

*"He calmed the storm to a whisper and stilled the waves. What a blessing was that stillness as he brought them safely into harbor!"* [1]

**Psalm 107:29, 30 (NLT)**

# STEADFAST

The day that I last saw Jenna in the hospital, a hospital worker asked me, "What is it about Jenna that makes her so special?" She had witnessed over a dozen of Jenna's friends and family come to see her in the hospital that day, all of us talking about how much we loved Jenna.

Once you met Jenna, you would understand why so many people cherished her. There was so much that made Jenna special.

Jenna really was one of the sweetest people you would ever meet. But she wasn't sweet for the sake of being sweet. Her sweetness came from a place of caring so very deeply for the people she loved. Her sweetness radiated from her because she so clearly reflected the Lord and His sweetness and love for us.

That last day in the hospital, as I walked into Jenna's hospital room, the first thing she did was ask about me. She wanted to know about what was going on in my life. That is who Jenna was. She was selfless and caring, wanting to hear how you were doing and how she could pray for you.

Jenna had been facing a tremendous amount of suffering at that point and had gone through so much in her journey with cancer. But through her suffering, we were able to witness how incredibly strong Jenna was. Her faith remained steadfast throughout her battle.

She, of course, had prayed that the cancer be taken from

her. But more than that, Jenna had prayed that her battle with cancer would point people to Christ.

The way Jenna endured this battle will forever stay with me. I saw tears and questions, doubts and fears, but ultimately, I saw Jenna draw even closer to the Lord. She trusted Him and the story He had written for her life. Her faith never wavered and she kept her eyes firmly focused on God and His promises to us.

Jenna really was so incredibly special.

*- Shannon S.*

# Dear Lord,

## - FLY YOUR BANNER HIGH -

## 05.07.16

*"Remember not the former things, nor consider the things of*
*old. Behold, I am doing a new thing; now it springs forth,*
*do you not perceive it? I will make a way in the wilderness,*
*rivers in the desert. The wild beasts will honor me, the jackals*
*and the ostriches, for I give water in the wilderness, rivers in*
*the desert, to give drink to my chosen people, the people whom*
*I formed for myself that they might declare my praise."* [1]
**Isaiah 43:18-21**

Jesus,

Thank you for laying this verse heavily on me today. I keep
saying how this time feels different. The situation we're in is

one I never even considered despite having cancer four times.

I pray you have big plans for this awfulness of a situation. I pray you use it to lift your name high. I think of all the people that could be touched by this because of the job you've given me, the places you've put me.

I ask again today, boldly, for complete healing. I praise you that you can do this and I praise you that it would obviously be you. I praise you for the people just now reading my blog. My family, my co-workers, and my friends who don't know you yet.

I pray you would shine bright and make them question. I pray they'd be attracted to you. I pray your goodness and grace and power would fly as a banner over us.

Go before us this weekend. Help us to love our family well. Move mountains, Lord. Kill all the cancer cells, dissolve them. I praise you for the incredible peace that has surrounded us the past few days. We are yours, Jesus. Do your thing here.

———

*"Behold, I am doing a new thing; now it springs forth,*

*do you not perceive it? I will make a way*

*in the wilderness, rivers in the desert."* [2]

**Isaiah 43:19**

# Dear Lord,

## - PEACE IN THE STORM -

## 05.09.16

Jesus,

My peace is directly correlated with time spent with you. I only gave you a little time yesterday and toward the end of the day, sadness and uncertainty were setting in. I thank you that you are my rock, my strength, and my peace.

Help Scott and I to keep our eyes on you, on our safe harbor. Keep our eyes set. I believe you are doing big things here. I believe you can (and I hope will) heal me. Either way, you are good and your plan is perfect.

I want to be around to tell of this great miracle you performed. Bring healing, Jesus.

Keep my eyes and ears open to hear and see you. Go before us. Do your thing. I praise you for the extra sweet moments you've given Scott and me.

I thank you for how pain knits closeness. We are yours, Jesus. Use us as you will, to bring praise to you and you alone. Amen.

————

*"Every word of God is flawless;*
*He is a shield to those who take refuge in Him."*
**Proverbs 30:5 (NIV)**

# Dear Lord,

## - WHILE ON VACATION -

## 05.30.16

Jesus,

Thank you for this beautiful place to relax and spend time with Scott and his family. It feels bittersweet because I keep thinking how this could be my last trip to Topsail Beach. I don't want to think like that, because I do believe you can heal, Jesus.

I also believe that you can heal me of this disease and impending death. Help Scott and I to squeeze close to you this week. Give us your presence, your peace, your words. I thank you for the sweet time we've had so far at the beach and it is only day 3.

I pray, Jesus, you'd keep us out of the hospital this week. Go before us. I pray you'd already be healing me of this cancer, bit by bit. Move in a big way, Lord. Help us to set our eyes on you, our safe harbor. Amen.

*"This is my comfort in my affliction,*
*that your promise gives me life."* [1]
**Psalm 119:50**

# RAINBOOTS

I had the privilege of doing life with Jenna when she married Scott and moved to Batesville. We were together for things related to Young Life (Club, Campaigners, and team meetings). We also met for a ladies Bible study with a few of our friends. And then there was church too! So yeah, I saw Jenna a lot and I had a chance to watch her life.

One of Jenna's favorite places was the hammock in their backyard where she would cuddle with the cat and read books. She often shared how she was encouraged or challenged in her faith by something she'd read in her latest book. She also created a warm and welcoming space by decorating their home with her art and photography.

She had time by herself—quiet time with her Lord when she prayed, interceded for family and friends, poured out her heart, and deepened her relationship with the Lord she loved. She was continually filled up with Christ and ready to pour Him out into the people around her.

I was intrigued. My life was packed full: a family, a full-time job, weekly Bible studies, and leadership roles in two wonderful ministries that I love! All these things were good things, but I found that my relationships were shallow.

I heard it said that God created us to be human beings, not human doings. Somehow, without my even realizing it, I had become a "doing."

Jenna's first priority was always Jesus and second was

201

people: loving them, listening to them, giving them the precious gift of time, speaking Words of Truth even when the circumstances were uncomfortable. For me, she was the living example of Ephesians 6:14-15, "Stand firm then, with the belt of truth buckled around your waist, with the breastplate of righteousness in place, and with your feet fitted with the readiness that comes from the Gospel of peace."

Because of her time spent with God, she was ready to speak words of Truth and Life. Because of her focus on the people around her, she had opportunities and boldness to do it!

At Jenna's funeral, I had an opportunity to look out on the faces that filled the church. Every seat was filled and people stood in the back. There were about 1,000 people there that evening. That memory is fixed in my mind and heart because God allowed me to see in those moments the impact of a life devoted to Christ.

Jesus, through Jenna, changed lives for eternity. I want to be used by God that way! I want that to be the legacy of my life!

I have a pair of Jenna's rain boots in a spot where I see them every day. They remind me to slow down my "doing," to rest, to spend time with my Lord, and then to run after those He loves.

"... and with your feet fitted with the readiness that comes from the Gospel of peace." [2]

*- Patti L.*

# Life since the bad news

## 06.07.16

So we kind of dropped a bomb here, then left you all hanging. That was unintentional. We have had a lot of peace since finding out, which is entirely the Holy Spirit. I've also noticed a very direct correlation with my time with Jesus and my attitude or outlook.

When I spend time with Him, I'm good and at peace. When I don't, my patience runs out really quick and I'm more likely to focus on the negative and be upset. Reminds me of the vision we got at Crossroads about keeping our eyes on the harbor and not on the storm.

It turns out that when you have cancer and it's not surgically removed, it hurts and is very uncomfortable. This is a first for me, because in the past they've always been able to take it out.

I've been seeing pain team to keep the pain and discomfort under control, which has been great, but also it has made me exhausted. I could sleep 24 hours a day and still be tired when I woke up. Scott keeps finding me sleeping, sitting up. They've also given me Ritalin to help me stay awake, so when there is a day I really want to be up and alert for, that has been helpful.

Along with the pain, another struggle has been shortness of breath. It is worst in the morning before my pain meds soak in. I move slowly. I told Scott I wasn't going to judge slow walkers anymore.

Right before we left for vacation they drained 650 mL of fluid off my right lung and that has helped tremendously. It helped with the shortness of breath, and also took away the pain I had when I hiccupped, which was bad enough that I had to yell out in pain.

The past 2 times we've had labs drawn, the tumor marker has leveled off and stayed the same, which is good. It was going up by 10 every time we had it drawn (weekly). We get more labs drawn tomorrow along with a CT to check on how much change there has been since the initial scans. We are obviously hoping for complete healing, but at least would like for it to be less or staying the same.

In other news, we are going to visit MD Anderson in Houston to see what options and trials they have available. We will call tomorrow to make an appointment.

They have been working closely with our doctors on my case, so we feel good about that, and we can rent a car and go visit Magnolia Market in Waco. So I'm pretty excited about that.

Our friends have started another page to help us out financially with another deductible around the corner, and travel expenses for our consult in Texas. and we are so blown away by everyone's generosity. If you gave, know that Scott and I could not thank you more. From the bottom of our hearts it means the world to us. It is one less stressor to worry about.

Speaking of that, you all have taken such good care of us as far as meals go. We have not had to worry about dinner for weeks now, and really haven't had to go to the grocery store. Which is especially great for Scott, because everything is sort of falling on him around here these days. He is the best. He serves me non-stop and without complaining. I am so blessed to be married to him.

One thing that repeatedly keeps showing up as a theme around here is that God has big plans up His sleeve. So many people, including those we know, and those who are just hearing our story for the first time, are telling us that God has pressed it on their hearts that God has healing in store here, and that this isn't the end.

We feel the same way. We are trusting Him for big things over here, and whichever way He chooses to answer our prayers for healing, He is still good.

In Daniel when the 3 Israelites were about to be thrown into the furnace they said,

*"If we are thrown into the blazing furnace, the God we serve is able to deliver us from it, and he will deliver us from Your Majesty's hand. But even if he does not, we want you to know, Your Majesty, that we will not serve your gods or worship the image of gold you have set up."* [1]
**Daniel 3:17, 18 (NIV)**

So we are over here, fully confident that God can and will heal. But in the same breath, if He chooses not to, we know He is good and that He loves us, so we can trust His plans, even if we hate that plan.

I just finished reading Tim Keller's book *Walking with God through Pain and Suffering,* and I have to recommend it to anyone who has ever struggled with the idea of suffering, or anyone that is walking through suffering themselves. One of the things he said, and I believe to the core of me is, "*Instead He gives us what we would have asked for if we had known everything He knows.*"

I know it seems like a stretch to say I'd ask for this, but it's also a stretch to say that I understand the unfolding of history better than He does. My favorite example was when he talked about Jesus hanging on the cross, what the people around watching must be thinking.

> "*But then, there you are at the cross with the few*
> *of his disciples who have the stomach to watch.*
> *And you hear people say, 'I've had it with this God.*
> *How could he abandon the best man we have ever seen?*
> *I don't see how God could bring any good out of this.*
>
> *What would you say? You would likely agree. And yet you are*
> *standing there looking at the greatest, most brilliant thing God*
> *could ever do for the human race.*" [2]

So that's about it for now over here. Please be praying for scans tomorrow, and pray for this coming weekend, we have a friend who is a part of a healing prayer ministry coming to pray over Scott and me. We know without a doubt that Jesus can heal, we are praying that He will.

Oh man, I can't not include this ... Scott and I went to the beach this past week, and while we were gone, two different friends showed up to surprisingly clean our house. The first was such a surprise, Scott didn't even know it was happening, so when my friend Shannon came, getting his approval, she showed up to a pretty clean house. But how sweet? She also stocked our freezer with meals (Thanks Shannon and Bob and Jeana and Owen!).

Then we got back home, and my old Bible study from Lexington came to hang out and love on me on Sunday. It was glorious. We just relaxed, talked, they made me delicious smoothies, they prayed for me, we all cried, and they drove all the way back to Lexington.

Thanks for sticking with this especially long update if you've made it this far!

———

*"There's a reason I am not writing the story and God is.*

*He knows how it all works out, where it all leads,*

*what it all means. I don't."* [3]

**Ann Voskamp**

# Dear Lord,

## - YOU MORE THAN ANYTHING -

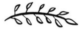

## 06.09.16

Jesus,

As you know, Scott and I got bad news yesterday. Tumor growth and the tumor marker has doubled.

I read an Oswald Chambers excerpt Scott sent me today, talking about sacrificing to get things from God, when God alone should be our desire. I feel torn about this because I don't think asking for you to heal me means I want healing more than I want you. If the only way to get healed meant life apart from you, I wouldn't want it, truly. I hope you know that, Jesus.

I want healing. I want to live my days here to point people to you. I want to stay with Scott. I know you can heal me.

BUT, if you explained the situation to me from what you know, and in that explanation, I would choose to not get healed, then I will trust you, because I know you only allow what will glorify you the most.

We will not stop crying out for your healing touch as long as we are here. Heal me as only you can, Jesus. Triumph over this cancer. We lay our lives before you, Jesus.

You are quite literally our only hope. In your sweet and powerful name I ask for healing. Draw Scott and me closer to you. In your name. Amen.

———

*"So we do not lose heart. Though our outer self is wasting away, our inner self is being renewed day by day. For this light momentary affliction is preparing for us an eternal weight of glory beyond all comparison, as we look not to the things that are seen but to the things that are unseen. For the things that are seen are transient, but the things that are unseen are eternal." [1]*

**2 Corinthians 4:16-18**

# Dear Lord,

## - HALF MY LIFE -

~~~~~~~~~~~~~~~

## 06.09.16

Jesus,

It has been 15 years.

Half my life has been spent walking with you, Jesus. I praise you for not letting me go. I thank you for holding tight to me.

I am at a low point today with a hard night last night and a new pain. This situation we're in feels more real and very threatening right now. Jesus, I ask you to heal.

If this cancer is not of you, you certainly can cause it to disappear. Heal me.

Thank you for an amazing husband who selflessly serves me non-stop. Draw us to your heart. We want you, Jesus.

I thank you for your faithfulness these 15 years and I ask that I'll still be walking with you in another 15. In your amazing and sweet name. Amen.

*"But those who die in the Lord will live; their bodies will rise again! Those who sleep in the earth will rise up and sing for Joy! For your life-giving light will fall like dew on your people in the place of the dead!"* [1]

**Isaiah 26:19 (NLT)**

# RESPONDING DIFFERENTLY

About five months after Jenna's passing, a very dreaded conversation happened within one of my patient's room. I had just accessed my patient's port and was cleaning up when the patient's mom asked about Jenna.

"Whatever happened to that one sweet nurse who battled cancer when she was younger? She has the cute dark hair with the pixie haircut. I'm pretty sure her name is Jenna. Did she leave, and go somewhere else to work? I hate to lose such an amazing nurse here on your team. We really miss her and haven't seen her in a while."

With my mask still on from the procedure, I turned to her with tears flowing down my face. My mask quickly became saturated from the tears as I was unable to hold back my uncontrollable grief. The patient's mom immediately noticed my reaction.

"What is it? What's wrong? Why are you crying?"

I gently delivered the news that Jenna had passed away the previous October after a long battle with ovarian cancer. I stood there with them as they experienced the devastation and shock upon hearing this news. They had no idea that Jenna, even as she cared for them, was sick herself.

"She mentioned she had cancer when she was younger, but never told us she was still fighting it."

The mom shared with me that Jenna was one of the most patient and kind nurses they ever had the pleasure to work with. As she processed what she had just heard, she began sharing a vivid memory of Jenna.

When Jenna was their nurse, she went to access her daughter's port for treatment, but missed the port (it was a very difficult port to access). It was in that moment where Jenna responded differently than anyone had before her.

Jenna sat beside her daughter on the bed, held her hand, and cried with her. As she sat with her, she quietly explained in her ever-loving, kind, and compassionate way that she knew exactly how she was feeling. She shared that she too had cancer when she was younger and knew the pain and anxiety of a port access.

The patient and mom went on to share the depth of how personal and comforting that moment was to them. That they had never experienced a nurse who was able to relate and connect on that level with her daughter. Ever since that moment, Jenna became one of their favorite nurses and they always hoped to get her whenever they came in for treatment or checkups.

Jenna never shared with them her current cancer diagnosis for a reason. She wanted them to see that she was a survivor, and that they too could overcome this.

*- Alicia H.*

# Treatment & life update

06.23.16

Hey everyone! So for the past 2 weeks I've said almost daily that I would write an update, and obviously failed, but not today! All credit probably goes to the 2 units of blood I got yesterday, giving me the energy for this.

So an update on where we are as far as treatment goes, if you could picture a list with numbered options of treatments on it, we are 3 down the list with 2 options crossed off.

Right now we are doing weekly Doxil, which is an IV chemotherapy, but thankfully, I haven't had any typical chemo side effects. We will add another med here soon that will be orally every day, with the fun side effect of turning my hair white (eek!). Please pray that these drugs would be stopping or slowing the cancer's growth enough to stay on it. The problems with the other things we've tried is that they weren't slowing it enough.

Since I reported in last, a lot has happened. I had another 900+ mL drained off my right lung, I had a 3-day inpatient stay to get my body used to TPN and lipids, so I could get IV nutrition every day at home. We did great with it in the hospital, but for whatever reason, when we got home and did it (it is an infusion that runs for 8 hours), it made me feel so awful. I threw up every time. So, we are going to try without the lipids and see if I can handle it better.

It would be a great load off if it would work, because it's 80% of my nutritional needs, and I need like 4,000 calories a day. With no appetite, that is impossible. So I guess another prayer request would be increased appetite/ability to eat and gain weight. I've lost around 20 lbs. since this all started, which is no good. Looking sickly over here.

We are still waiting on MD Anderson in Texas to call with an appointment, which should be any day now, so I'll try to keep you posted on that.

Yesterday was chemo #2, and we were all ready to go home after, when we learned my hemoglobin was 7, and that I would have to stay to get 2 units of blood. So we ended up being at the hospital for almost 12 hours yesterday, yuck.

On our way home Scott let me pick up a pizza, and when we pulled off to get it, we got a flat tire in the parking lot. Our sweet new kitten had been home all day by herself in the laundry room, we were so sad. I have a co-worker that thankfully lives right by there that came to the rescue. Scott patched the tire and put it on with the help of her hubby, and we finally made it home.

Oh yeah, you read right. Scott bought a kitten! She's the tiniest thing ever (can sit on my regular iPhone 6), and so sweet. Her name is Waffles.

In other news, my co-workers threw a benefit dinner for me on Monday night at Frida in Covington. It was amazing. They all organized baskets to raffle off, the food was incredible, the entire restaurant voluntarily opened just for us. They also donated $1,000.

People, seriously go eat there. It's adorable, amazing food, the sweetest area, you have to go support them. I think the benefit raised over $6,000. So, thank you so much to everyone who came and who made it happen. Scott and I are so blown away.

On that note, I'll post a video because typing words won't do justice, and we can't possibly write thank you notes to everyone who has supported us financially through our "GoFundMe" page, or just sent checks in. There are hundreds of you, literally. So please, if that's you, watch the video! [1]

This morning I listened to an old Rend Collective album, and the song "My Lighthouse" [2] came on, and I almost couldn't believe I didn't connect the dots sooner. So many people have cast this vision over Scott and I of steering a boat into harbor outrunning a storm, and this song is so perfect for that vision, and so encouraging. It was so good for my heart this morning. Just a reminder He is going before and behind us, and because of that we can face each day full of peace.

Y'all, one last thing. For my birthday, Scott let me order wood signs from my friend Angie. She has an Etsy shop, Thirsty Heart Designs, that is incredible. She specialized in hand-lettered items. So we gave Angie a couple of our favorite verses in Isaiah, and she wove them together and delivered our signs yesterday.

Thanks for sticking with me. Love you all. Thank you for praying. Jesus is our only hope right now, and while it's a sad and hard situation, it really is a blessing for Him to be all we have. Because we know in that, that He is all we need.

*"It is the Lord who goes before you. He will be with you;*
*he will not leave you or forsake you. Do not fear or be dismayed."*[3]

**Deuteronomy 31:8**

# Dear Lord,

## - GLIMPSES OF YOU -

July 2016

Jesus,

I thank you for feeling great yesterday and what a gift that was. I thank you for new life that has sprung up all around.

Help us to encourage and disciple well. I lift up healing today, Jesus. Please remove this cancer. Every last cell. I know you can Jehovah Rapha, and I thank you for that.

I pray also that those in my life would get a glimpse of you by knowing and watching our story play out. Help us to be light and salt. In your holy and sweet name. Amen.

---

*"Don't begrudge the difficult days. I know they're hard.*
*Don't Hate them. God's at work in the mess."* [1]

**Matt Chandler**

# RESILIENT LIGHT

I had the privilege of living with Jenna for two and a half years while we attended the University of Kentucky. Jenna was and remains to this day, the sweetest person I have ever met. All of us roommates—myself, Shannon, Emily, Kyle, and Jeana—celebrated Jenna whenever something good came her way.

It was impossible to be jealous of Jenna because it truly seemed that she deserved every last ounce of goodness in the world. We cheered her on when she applied for nursing school and rejoiced for her when she received her acceptance letter (and other things like her car and MacBook).

I will always remember Jenna's brightly colored study notes and how she wrote with skinny Crayola markers whenever possible. Everything about Jenna was bright and happy. Even her dryer lint was sometimes pink because of how much she wore bright colors.

Despite being extremely busy with nursing school, Jenna always made time for what mattered most—God first and people second. She had a relationship with her Lord and Savior like I had never seen before. She poured over Scripture and was always reading a Christian book as well.

I remember her love for C. S. Lewis, *The Ragamuffin Gospel* by Brennan Manning, and the Christian fiction novel *Redeeming Love* by Francine Rivers. She devoured that book and told everyone how much we needed to read it.

For some reason, it took me until 2016 (ten years after we lived together and the year Jenna passed) to get around to reading it, and I could immediately see why it captivated Jenna's heart. It's a love story based on the book of Hosea that mirrors the unending love the Father has for his bride, the church.

The "bride" in the story is actually very troubled and rebellious, not at all the good Christian girl you might expect. Jenna understood that at our core we are all deeply flawed sinners deserving of death. We are lost and hopeless without the redeeming love of our Savior.

While I often strived to prove myself worthy of the Father's love, Jenna was always so humble about who she was and everything she had been given. She knew that everything in this life is a gift.

Everything about Jenna was joyful and attractive in the sense that you wanted to be around her. Every time I interacted with her, I left happier and encouraged. She had a light about her that we all knew was a direct result of her relationship with God.

She was radiant and shined wherever she went, just like Moses did after descending Mount Sinai. While I'll never understand why God took Jenna at such a young age, I know that the impact she made during her short time on Earth was immense. I am forever grateful that I had the opportunity to know her and live with her for just that short amount of time.

*- Tiffany P.*

# Dear Lord,

## - SHINE THROUGH -

---

## July 2016

Jesus,

I am grateful today for you. I am grateful you sent me words I needed as I needed them. I need you to show up where I'm stuck, Jesus.

I pray non-stop for healing, but want to have my eyes open to all the ways you want to use this sickness. I know you have plans, even for mundane days.

I ask that you'd help me to love and be a light to everyone at the hospital you have placed on my heart and in my path. Help me to have a servant's heart when I'm there—especially on the hard days.

Help me, above all, to keep my eyes set on you. Help me to take my focus off of myself throughout the day and seek what you have for me. In your holy and sweet name. Amen.

*"... Laughter does not exclude weeping. Christian joy is not an escape from sorrow. Pain and hardship still come, but they are unable to drive out the happiness of the redeemed."* [1]

**Eugene Peterson**

# HARD TO LOVE

I met Jenna for the first time when I was a freshman in high school. She was a sophomore in college and led Young Life at my school. I will never forget the day I walked out of the school and met her in the parking lot, talking to a group of my friends.

Immediately two thoughts went through my head—*One, what are you doing in a high school parking lot!? And two, what are you so dang happy about!?* But Jenna kept showing up ... to the parking lot, to the lunch room, to the student section of the football game. The more I was around her, the more I kept noticing that there was definitely something different about this girl.

She was kind and gentle, always smiling, always laughing (silently), and always so full of joy. And though as a lost, broken, and hurting 14-year-old girl, I would have never admitted it, and certainly never acted like it, I adored Jenna from the start.

However, I certainly did not make it easy on her! I was the definition of hard to love—bitter, cynical and stubborn as can be. I could tell story after story of the hard time I gave sweet Jenna. More than once I left an inappropriate comment on her Facebook wall such as "Thanks for buying us all that alcohol, Jenna, you're the best!" Or there was the time my friends and I baked Jenna a "Happy National Cheer up the Lonely Day" cake and left it on her front porch in a rather obnoxious manner. We banged on the door repeatedly until Jenna, sure someone was breaking in, called the cops in a panic. When the cops showed up we were long gone, but the cake was still there, and the cops promptly asked Jenna, *"Are you lonely?"*

That may have been the closest I ever got to seeing Jenna angry. Seriously, I was the worst! Despite how challenging I was, Jenna never gave up on me, and she never gave up on me knowing Jesus.

She had this vision for what my life could be in Christ and she was so confident that the Lord would see it to fruition. She boldly and faithfully pursued me until one day, as a junior in high school, I finally came face to face with my need for a Savior.

As I surrendered my life to Christ and began walking with Him, she held the crown above my head and she helped me grow into it. She taught me how to love God's Word, how to pray, how to share the Gospel, and so much more. But more than anything, she taught me that Jesus was IT, that even in pain and suffering and brokenness and yes, even cancer, that He was absolutely and undoubtedly it, that He was enough for her and enough for me.

Because of that, because of the way Jenna leveraged her life, I have been radically and eternally changed.

At Jenna's celebration, I had the privilege of standing on stage and telling everyone in the room how knowing Jenna had changed my life. At the end, I asked for people to stand if Jenna had impacted them and their walk with Jesus as well. As I stood on stage, I watched nearly half of the room stand. I will never forget that moment.

In that moment, I had never been so sure in Jesus, I had never been so sure that He really is it, and I had never been so sure that life truly is found in giving ours away. I will never stop telling people about sweet Jenna. But more importantly, I will never stop telling people about Jesus because of Jenna.

- *Katie L.*

# Dear Lord,

## - EVERYONE MUST KNOW -

## 07.26.16

Jesus,

I thank you for truth and focus that were both much needed this morning. I loved 2 Corinthians 4. In verse 12 it says, *"so death is at work in us, but life in you."* [1]

There is so much applicable about this passage in this season of life, Jesus. I am physically wasting away. I pray I would carry around your death so that everyone I come in contact with could experience your life.

I know there are (most) days when I turn inward and am caught up in my own world of sadness, but help me to remember to tell your story with my life.

I pray for our appointment today at MD Anderson, that the doctors would have helpful information for us, some treatment options. I still am praying for healing, Jesus. Go before us Lord. I'm sorry for being bratty yesterday.

Take over my heart, mind, and words today. In your Son's amazing name, amen.

———

*"Knowing that he who raised the Lord Jesus*
*will raise us also with Jesus and bring us*
*with you into his presence."* [2]
**2 Corinthians 4:14**

# FOR ONE KID

Being a Young Life leader requires sacrifice. It requires you to be selfless. Young Life leaders build relationships with kids and walk alongside them through the ups and downs of life. You don't get to just show up once a week to a program. It takes investment and intentionality. Year after year. Month after month. Week after week. Day in and day out.

As Jenna's condition grew worse, I wanted her to know that she was welcome to choose to be a part of anything she wanted to be a part of and to stay home when she felt like it was too much. On most days, Jenna chose to be present, even in the midst of her pain and weakness. She chose to share her story and to be vulnerable.

The summer before Jenna passed away, we were gearing up for our summer trip with kids. I wanted Jenna to know that it was completely up to her if she wanted to go on the trip. It was becoming very apparent that things were becoming much more difficult for her. At the same time, I knew how much Jenna absolutely loved taking girls to Young Life Camp.

Jenna spent four years chasing after a specific girl, trying to get her to camp. It was four years of relationship building, four years of texting and long conversations about life, four years of praying. At times, I'm sure it seemed like all of the effort was going nowhere.

Then something miraculous happened. After those four years, the high school girl Jenna had been pouring her life into decided to go. Jenna was determined to experience that week with her, and so she went, following the bus along the way in her car as Scott drove.

When we arrived at camp, Jenna drove a golf cart around camp to watch her high school friend experience an unforgettable week. There were times when Jenna would lay on the floor before events as she dealt with pain and discomfort. Yet, not once did she ever complain. She wanted to be there for her high school friend. I remember thinking, "*I work for this organization, and if I was in Jenna's shoes, I don't think I would have gone on this trip.*"

Jenna had a different perspective on life, though. She had clarity. She knew what was important. She knew what would last and what wouldn't. She had her hope in Jesus and her eyes fixed on eternity.

Jenna had faith in Jesus. And not the kind of faith that just helps you feel good about life or helps you sleep better at night. She had the kind of faith I can only hope and pray to have. She had the kind of faith and trust in Jesus that moved her to believe it's worth any amount of pain and suffering for others to have the opportunity to know life with Him. And I know she would say it was all worth it.

Even if it was just for one kid.

*- Sean B.*

# Dear Lord,

## - FOCUS MY HEART -

## July 2016

Jesus,

I pray today that your glory would be my focus. In all that I do, or say. Help me to not think about my own self, but you and how the world sees you.

Go before me as I disciple today. Give me your Spirit's words and prompts. Help me to take time deep and get to the heart of where you want to be with her.

I thank you for my sweet husband who strives to make my dreams come true. Bless him so so much. In your name, I give myself to you, Jesus. Amen.

*"We have the Spirit of God IN us. People are reading*
*our lives. We may be the only Bible someone ever reads."*
**a note from Jenna next to 2 Corinthians 3:2, 3**

*"You yourselves are our letter of recommendation, written*
*on our hearts, to be known and read by all. And you showed*
*that you are a letter from Christ delivered by us, written not*
*with ink but with the Spirit of the living God, not on*
*tablets of stone but on tablets of human hearts."* [1]
**2 Corinthians 3:2, 3**

# SOMETHING GREATER

As I drove out of the hospital parking lot, I saw the most beautiful sunset. It was as if to say, "The darkness cannot drown out **this** light."

And Oh, it has not.

I have always known Jenna was set apart. She was kinder, softer, more joyful than most. She loved Jesus with a passion and persistence that seemed untamable. It seemed wild.

I mean, this past summer she chose to go to Young Life camp as a leader with her girls, in the midst of chemo and cancer for the fourth round to give one more word, one more push towards Jesus. Her life screamed of her lavish love towards her heavenly father.

The world could look on her story of cancer since high school and think, "How are you the way you are?" To look at her joy made you look inward and ask yourself, "What does Jenna understand, that I do not?" Oh God, if I could be half the woman that Jenna was, I would be honored.

But as I left the hospital for the last time, it clicked. Jenna has always understood Jesus in a way that most of us never have. She understood heaven. She understood that we live in the "valley of the shadow of death." She understood and lived out the truth that our God is our husband, with an unfailing love that will never leave us or forsake us. It will not diminish with age, it does not run out, it does not perish.

As the Apostle, Paul says, *"to live is Christ, to die is to gain."*[2] I am now understanding that this was our Jenna's mindset. And what that produced was one of the most loving, intentional women I have ever met.

I had the privilege of shepherding her high school girls that she led to Christ when they came to college. Year after year, I have called Jenna for counsel when I felt like my sin, my junk was screwing them up, or when I had no idea what I was doing, or how to speak correct truth into their lives. She was a soft and firm place to land. Her words were soaked in wisdom and her understanding was more gracious than my hardened heart could ever comprehend.

As I sit here and write out these words and think of the hundreds of memories, I am overwhelmed at the realization that Jenna was the closest earthly image of Jesus that I have ever seen. Rightly so, she walked close to Him faithfully.

We sat in the waiting room of the hospital and listened to stories of Jenna and we heard her father tell us of the first time she got on the bus to go to YL camp in the midst of her first round of cancer.

I kept thinking in my head, God used the darkest place in her life to bring her to Him. What Satan intended for evil, God made good.

Oh, and He made so much good out of Jenna's life. There were not enough shadows or darkness to hide the light that came forth on that day. If she were here now, she would tell me to tell you that Jesus is absolutely it.

From beginning to end, Jenna's life was so very important. Important, because it reminds us that this life is hard and no one is exempt from death. Important, because her life reminds us that this place is not our home. Important, because her life reminds us that there is something Greater for us.

"*Where, O death, is your victory? Where, O death, is your sting?*" [3] Death does not have the victory here. Why? Because Jenna is healed and whole and feasting with our faithful, unfailing Father.

Someday, I will sit at the table with her again. Jenna spent her whole life telling others about the only one who gives her Life. "*His love is better than life*" she would say. And I am here to tell you that was what she echoed even into her last days. Especially in her last days.

Now, I realize I may never be as sweet as Jenna. That is pretty freaking hard to compete with. But man, will I echo her joy and love for her Savior until my final days as well? And so goes the list of every person who encountered Jenna, who by default, had a taste of our sweet Jesus. Job well done, Jenna. We promise to pick up our slack in your honor. Heavenward, I say.

*- Angie P.*

# Long update & Young Life camp

## 08.03.16

I am the worst updater! I apologize. I can't tell you how many times I thought about sitting down to write, and just kept putting it aside. So much since I last checked in!

Treatment wise, we're still doing the weekly Doxil (IV chemo in the hospital) and now the oral Pazopanib daily. We will be doing scans here soon to check on how effective this has been.

If it is effective (slowing the growth or shrinking it), we'll continue on these. If it is not effective, we will move to a couple immune therapy drugs (if insurance will allow it in my case). So that will be a big prayer request should we need to move to the next option. These drugs aren't typically used in cases like mine, so it may be a fight to get them. Still feeling good with the weekly chemo, which is great.

July has been CRAZY! We've been to 4 states, traveling every weekend. We are excited to stay home for a bit this month.

The first weekend of July we went to Philadelphia for a wedding. Our Young Life teammates' daughter got married, and they rented out a B&B (it was to die for). They gave us what I'm pretty sure was the master bedroom there (way too sweet of them), and just let us hang out and enjoy for a few days. It was so perfect.

We relaxed a bit with our sweet friends there for a few days, and on the last day, when we all left, we headed to New Jersey with our friends the Boyces and the Bohls.

We went to a sweet little town that I lived in during 7th grade. I grew up in NJ basically from 1989-1999, so the one year living in this town doesn't compare with the almost 10 years of north Jersey, but if you've ever been to Spring Lake, you'd understand why we chose it.

It is right on the shore, and full of gorgeous giant homes, a sweet little main street with candy shops and pizzerias. Turns out it was $10 per person to go on the beach (?!), but we hung out on the boardwalk and walked around. I brought them for slices of pizza and then Italian ice in a neighboring town before we headed back to Pennsylvania.

The next 2 weekends were traveling to and from Young Life camp. My favorite week of the year!

Scott and I drove behind the bus so I could recline and sleep on the way there and back. In short, it was an amazing week. I had to stay in a room separate from the high school girls, and had a little golf cart to get around quickly, so it looked a little different than other years leading, but was still great.

I essentially went for one girl going, which made it really relaxing and awesome. We had the sweetest cabin of girls ever, who wanted to spend all their free time together and threw gummy bears up on the ceiling until they stuck. Love them.

We got to dive into who Jesus is, and what He offers us. We got to have intentional and deep conversation every day with our high school friends. Which is the best thing in the world, if you ask me. We got to see some sweet friends walk over from death to life, and I just felt so thankful to be allowed to be a part of this amazing thing God is doing in hearts.

This past weekend we went to Houston, Texas for a consult with doctors at MD Anderson. We had to spend thousands of dollars to essentially talk to a doctor for 30 minutes, and while that is frustrating, it's good we went and had that conversation.

Texas is HOT. I will not ever live there. I don't know how anyone does. Scott and I spent a lot of time napping in our air-conditioned hotel room.

The first day there was just travel, the second day we waited 3 hours to see a doctor for 5 minutes, and the third day we finally had a helpful conversation with the doctor. So we reported back to our doctor, and the next day we went to Waco (FIXER UPPER!!!!)!

We got to see Common Grounds, a little coffee shop that one of the first season couples own. We went to Clint's store (Harp Designs), and his house is right next door, which was one of my favorite fixer uppers they ever did.

Then Scott and I headed over to the silos where Magnolia Market is, as well as the bakery, the seed and supply shop, outdoor lawn games, food trucks, and basically everything beautiful.

Scott informed me that our friends set up a little private tour (so sweet!), so we got to go up to see the offices and got a bird's-eye-view of all that was happening on the grounds. I got some pretty things, and before I died of heat, we left and headed to catch our plane in Houston. Whirlwind!

So now we are home, I got some more Doxil yesterday (by yesterday I mean almost a week ago; I almost finished this post, then pressed pause for a bit).

Our sweet kitten is growing, but still seems so tiny to me. She is so sweet, loves rubbing her face against ours.

I've been feeling so much better than a month or so ago. I'm moving around on my own better, haven't had any shortness of breath (or fluid drained for that matter). I still have other annoying issues with my body not functioning normally, one of which is my low appetite and weight loss. I'm debating talking to the doctors about getting a feeding tube in my stomach so I can get feeds throughout the day to try to reach my calorie goal. I have got to stop losing weight. I feel like I look scary.

As far as prayer goes, we'd love prayer that the Doxil and Pazopanib would be working, pray still for full healing, pray for appetite and weight gain. Pray that Scott and I would be leaning in hard to Jesus. I know this season holds a lot of growth and closeness to Him if we'd allow it.

A few random things, I recently celebrated my 15 years since I began a relationship with Jesus, which, now that I'm 30, is half my life! Crazy.

It's so awesome to watch how faithful He has been. I had no idea when I set out, the adventure He'd have ahead, but man I'm so thankful for a God that never leaves us or forsakes us.

I read Psalm 119:50 the other day, and it says

*"This is my comfort in my affliction,*
*that your promise gives me life."* [1]

I love that having life is not mutually exclusive from affliction. Just knowing Jesus gives life in any situation. I'd take Him and all this craziness over perfect health without Him any day.

Last thing! Sorry! I read this in Jennie Allen's *Restless* the other day and felt called out and challenged. She is talking about her friend who is in a coma with young kiddos at home and asking God why.

Did He forget about her? Forget how much she loves Him? That her kids need her? She was walking in the lobby of the hospital (by a cross statue) and heard God say to her the following:

*"I have forgotten nothing. And I am not passive about my approach to this problem. I deal. I deal with this sickness and pain and death. I do not forget. I bleed out for this.*

*So as you walk past me on that cross, Jennie, into a room that feels out of control and full of suffering, don't see a weak, distant, forgetful God.*

*You see a God who tells oceans where to stop and a God who tells evil where to stop. You see a God who bleeds out for those you hurt for. You see a God who suffered first. I AM with you. And I have a plan here."* [2]

Just real good stuff. I love that God weeps and mourns with us. That He walked the path of suffering first so I could look to Him for comfort.

To leave on a really fun note, our sweet wedding photographer, Cara Dee, offered recently to give us the proceeds from her mini sessions, which is the sweetest, but on top of that, she said she'd be passing through our little town, and would love to take our pictures as well.

We got our photos in the mail the other day and basically love every last one of them, but if you're from Lexington, hire her to snap your pics!

*"In this last summer of her life, one of the last major things she did was take students to camp. It blows me away. No matter where she was in her fight, her battle with cancer, she continued to be creative and faithful. She continued to be hopeful and excited for a life with Jesus."* [3]

**Justin Ryder, Young Life Staff and Podcast**

# CELEBRATIONS

celebrate /sel-*uh*-breyt/ *verb* **1** to rejoice in or have special festivities to mark (a happy day, event, etc.) **2** to observe (a day) or commemorate (an event) with ceremonies or festivities **3** to make known publicly; proclaim

When I think of Jenna, I think of how she loved to celebrate. All kinds of things. Big and small. Holidays, babies, seasons, anniversaries, birthdays, cats, weddings, accomplishments, people, milestones, new movies or books, the return of a television show. You name it, it could have a reason to be celebrated in Jenna's mind. Any excuse for people to be together, she was all for it. Any excuse to make someone feel special, she was excited about it and wanted to make it happen.

One of my favorite memories with Jenna (and our friends) was when we road-tripped to Philadelphia in July of 2016 to celebrate a friend's wedding. We all stayed in a rental house together, ate, reminisced, and laughed a lot. Jenna never once complained on that trip despite her physical condition. But I saw a glimpse of how difficult it was for her to be in a car that long, to not be in her own home, to struggle finding something to eat because she had lost her appetite, to be around so many people, to fight the exhaustion her body couldn't let go of. Jenna had every excuse to skip out on this celebration, but she wouldn't. That wasn't her.

God commands us to celebrate. I think this is probably because He knows that we often get caught up on ourselves, life's circumstances and situations. When we're busy, we struggle to celebrate. When we feel we're drowning in brokenness, despair, and helplessness; we struggle to celebrate. It is human nature for us to focus on the bad.

To celebrate requires faith. To celebrate requires action. It requires us to follow through. Celebration is relational—something Jenna was all about. It requires us to stop, rest, and shift priorities. This is often counter-cultural in our world today. To celebrate takes effort, often it can even require sacrifice. It helps us shift our perspective off of us and onto God. It ultimately reminds us of God's goodness, something Jenna never forgot.

It amazes me how even in her last days on Earth, Jenna was focused on the celebration that would take place in heaven, not her current circumstances.

Even after Jenna's life on Earth ended, the goal and hope was to celebrate her. There wasn't a funeral or memorial service. Instead there was a celebration of her life.

- *Kelsey B.*

# Scans and the plan

## 08.25.16

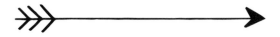

W hat a week! Scott and I started the week out with the Great Darke County Fair, which is the only way to start off a week. If you've never been, you need to find a way to go. It's in his hometown of Greenville, Ohio and it's nothing short of wonderful. I got pushed in a wheelchair along with all the old ladies, and got to eat all the great fair food.

Tuesday rolled around and that meant scans. I got a CT scan, and we found out yesterday at our chemo appointment that the tumor in my abdomen has grown more than they'd like to see, but the one on my lung has stayed the same, which is good.

We were expecting this, although I have been feeling "good" lately, so we wouldn't have been surprised if there were no growth either. I say "good" because I have been feeling "good" lately, but my good is not the same as your average person. My good usually means I still move super slowly and can't walk very far without tuckering out, along with stomach discomfort.

So, yesterday we did not get our regularly planned chemo, but moved on to the next treatment plan, which involves immunotherapy.

We will get Pembrolizumab IV once every 21 days, and I believe that will be an overnight inpatient stay in order to get it approved by insurance. This is an immunotherapy used mainly for melanoma and lung cancers.

There are a few hurdles to why we don't feel great about this drug in my case, but it has been used in random tumors before and done really well. It's never been tested with my type of tumor, so I'm hoping mine will be one it works well with.

A prayer request would be that my body would find a reason for this drug to target my cancer cells. The second immunotherapy med I will get, we started yesterday. That is Azacitidine, which is a subQ injection in the skin for 7 days, then off for 28 days.

This drug will wake up cells my body hasn't used since it was an embryo in hopes that my body will recognize my tumor as foreign. The Azacitidine hopefully will act as an enhancer to the Pembrolizumab. So we will give this combo a few months to do its thing and then scan to see what is happening. The goal of these meds isn't for the tumor to stay the same, but to shrink. So pray for that.

We also found out yesterday that when my short-term disability turns into long-term, I lose my status as employee, which means I lose my insurance. This is a BIG DEAL. That switch happens October 2nd.

We just finished our out of pocket costs for this cycle (July-June), so it's especially sad to have to figure out what to do about insurance. We're looking into everything. I would even do paperwork at home to stay an employee if they'd let me. I don't know what we'll do and I'm pretty sure Scott is stressed, but I do know that God will take care of it. He always does. So I'm resting in that.

The really great thing about yesterday is after such a crazy day full of stressful news, I got to go straight to a fancy spa with a sweet co-worker to get fancy agave nectar pedicures.

One of the care managers at work gave my co-worker a gift card for us two to go get pampered, and it was absolutely the most perfect thing that could have happened. I haven't had a pedicure in 15 years, I'm pretty sure, and let me tell you, I love them.

This place (The Woodhouse Day Spa in Kenwood), was so fancy. I walked in and they offered me a drink and took me to a relaxation room while I waited for Annie. Then we went back to the pedicure room where I got to sit in a fancy massage chair with warm things around my neck and my feet in warm water. I wasn't even too ticklish! Oh man. It was perfection. Thank you so so much for that amazing generosity (you know who you are).

In other news, girl trip to Harry Potter world is up and running smoothly for now. We have 15 girls going, so watch out, Orlando. Please be praying that I'll still feel good when that rolls around at the end of September.

Scott and I are taking a day at a time over here, so we're doing pretty good. God's Word keeps proving to be exactly what I need to hear when I need to hear it. It's funny, Scott can tell the days I spend time with Jesus in the morning versus the days I don't (embarrassed money emoji would go here).

This morning was really sweet when I was reading 2 Corinthians. In 1:9-10 it says,

*"Indeed, we felt that we had received the sentence of death.*
*But that was to make us rely not on ourselves but on*
*God who raises the dead. He delivered us from*
*such a deadly peril, and he will deliver us.*

*On him we have set our hope that he will deliver us again.*
*You also must help us by prayer, so that many will give*
*thanks on our behalf for the blessing granted*
*us through the prayers of many."* [1]

The paragraph right before it was all about God's comfort for us in our trials. The Word of God is literally alive and active, and I am so thankful for that. He always gives me what I need when I show up to listen.

That's about it over here. To recap, we need prayer that these new immunotherapy drugs would work against this tumor, as well as for insurance to work out somehow (preferably without Scott having to get a job that won't allow him to be with me).

And, as always, for healing. Whether that be through these drugs or straight up God, we'll take whatever. But mostly that our eyes would be set on Jesus. We love you all! Thanks for following along and for praying.

———

*"Purge me with hyssop, and I shall be clean; wash me and I shall*
*be whiter than snow. Let me hear joy and gladness;*
*let the bones that you have broken rejoice."* [2]

**Psalm 51:7, 8**

# WAND OF VALOR

My thoughts vacillated. What can I do? What is there to do? Should I do something? I landed on doing something. Something for Jenna, something with thought, something with care. Something to make her feel loved. Some tiny element of surprise. Doesn't Jenna love surprises?

Several of us did something. Some planned details for the momentous trip to Harry Potter World. Some thought up and designed a group "Gilfendor" T-shirt. Some paid for all of the shirts for twenty of our girlfriends. Some bought plane tickets or drove across states just to be present.

I finally landed: I commissioned a friend to make fifteen individual Harry Potter wands. I would distribute them at the hotel in Orlando. This was my something.

As the weekend approached, our girlfriends started visiting Jenna that last week in the hospital. Jenna wouldn't be making the trip. We gathered in the waiting room, taking turns to visit her in pairs. I distributed the wands. It wasn't the perfect thing to do or to have; it was just my something.

Each wand was in a personalized sleeve, with its own Latin name, based on the owner's most prevalent quality. Surrounding each girl's name were several additional qualities that I see in her.

Such a diversity of steadfast friends' personalities was read. It was my hope that each wand served as a physical symbol of those sweet moments we were privileged to share with valiant Jenna.

*Jenna*
*Baculum Valorsum: Wand of Valor*

Valiant, peace bearer, temperate, assured, merciful, hospitable, truth speaker, reliable, fearless, perceptive, speaker of hope, imaginative, serene, dreamer, empathetic

Isn't she valiant? The word is reminiscent of the Narnia series, where a girl knows that there is a world beyond what eyes can see, and she gets to experience it before the others, earning the epithet Queen Lucy, the Valiant. As she rested her head on the pillow, Jenna flicked her wand back and forth, and listened to us read her qualities.

I know she was encouraged; I flash back to a favorite passage of the transfiguration when Moses and Elijah encouraged Jesus before His death. What a privilege to be her encourager: valiant Jenna, living before all of us in the world that our eyes can't yet see.

*– Lucianne J.*

# Dear Lord,

## - ONE LAST ENTRY -

$$\textit{ffff}$$

## 09.07.16

Jesus,

I feel like I have not spent time crying out to you lately. We've kind of adopted a living in the present mentality, which means not giving a lot of thought to this situation as a whole and I feel like in order to deal with it (I know I need to because emotions are so close to the surface). I need to be crying out to you more. It will allow me to deal and draw me to your heart. So help lead me in that.

When it comes down to it, I think I am expecting the worst, but not acknowledging it. I don't want to expect you to not heal me because I know you can. And I know your timing looks a lot different than mine. So help me to keep my mind and heart open for the miracle that I know you can do.

Anyway, help me to start the process of digging into this hard situation we're in. Allow me to deal with it healthily and in a way that binds me even closer to you.

Be with Scott and be building him into yourself. I pray he'd be leaning on you and not on his own two feet. Show me how to love and encourage him best. I thank you that you hold the reins. In your holy and good and powerful name I place this in your hands and at your feet. Amen.

———

*"The one thing I ask of the Lord—the thing I seek most—is to live in the house of the Lord all the days of my life, delighting in the Lord's perfections and meditating in his Temple."* [1]

**Psalm 27:4 (NLT)**

# HOPE IN DARK DAYS

I was in over my head with chemical depression. Life piled on top of depression and depression piled on top of life. And there I was, buried.

Then, a miscarriage. The miscarriage was painfully slow. First, we found out there was no longer a heartbeat. Then we waited on my body to get the message. But it wasn't getting the message.

I had to take medication to expedite the process. The night I took the medication, half-conscious on pain meds, we got a phone call that Jenna likely wouldn't make it through the night.

Dear God.

The world held onto Jenna for several days. My body held onto that lost baby for several more.

Dark days. Sad days.

On my dresser, I placed Jenna's joyful photo next to my ultrasound picture. Two gifts. Two losses. Looking at them side by side, it struck me that they were together. I don't know how it all works in heaven, but when I imagined that the Jenna we lost might be mothering the baby we lost—I felt hope.

No one better to take care of a precious gift, than a precious gift. I rest in that.

*- Andrea V.*

# The last battle

## 01.17.17

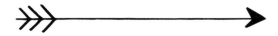

Much has happened since the last update in August, but I feel as though Jenna's story has too much to offer to let it sit idle in my mind. And though I will skip a lot of the details, it is my hope that you will experience both Jesus and Jenna as you continue reading.

Also, make sure you give me a little grace, as we all know that Jenna was a far superior and far more inspirational writer. As for the title, it comes directly from Jenna as she told me in her last week that it was a book I HAD to read (and which I did read; *The Last Battle*—The Chronicles of Narnia by C. S. Lewis)

The month of September brought a lot of hard days. Mentally for me; physically for Jenna. More and more often she felt ill, and many days she could only lay in a ball on the couch to ease the pain.

Yet, throughout all of it, she never complained. We still had full confidence in complete healing from the Lord. As the days and weeks moved forward, good days were fewer and farther to come by. My heart took a beating that month as I could literally do nothing to ease the pain of my wife. All I could do was bring her things she needed and sit with her as she battled the pain.

Looking back now, I cherish these moments.

And yet, even as good days diminished, she fully expected to go Harry Potter World at the end of September. The plan was for a 5-day Nutritional in-patient stay at Cincinnati Children's Liberty to get her energy and nutrition up, and then be on her way with her wonderful Lexington friends to Orlando.

To say she was excited would be selling it short.

And so, we packed our bags and headed for our in-patient stay. To make things even better, our doctor (whom we love) was on service at the Liberty campus that week. It all seemed perfect to set us out for new adventures.

The first few days went as planned. Jenna received nutrition, and I ran a few errands in Cincinnati a little each day—we all know how much I needed to get out of the hospital to stay cheerful.

Our plan only took us as far as those first few days. Beyond that, I came face to face with the realization that the world is out of my hands. As much control as I wanted to have or thought I had, I learned quickly and painfully that this world doesn't always respond to my plans, my wants, or my hopes.

Day 3 or 4, I'm not exactly sure, brought news that I've dreaded since we started walking down this road again. The pain she was having wasn't caused by any fluid (which we were hoping). The pain was, in fact, coming from a partially obstructed bowel caused by ever-expanding cancer tissue. This, an inoperable, no solution scenario. And so we could only wait. Dreadfully wait.

By the time I came to realize what this actually meant, Jenna was already being heavily sedated at her request to minimize the pain. This meant that our conversations became very short-lived as she slept more often. As the week went by, many of our dear friends and family came to see Jenna. To say their goodbyes. To comfort me.

My heart aches as I re-live these experiences for the first time as I write this. But these tears are good tears; tears of loss, but tears of joy and cleansing.

To watch the lives of those she impacted show up that week was beauty in a pit of despair. To see Jenna when she was awake inquire about the lives of those who visited, while deflecting her own condition, showed her heart and her love for others beyond herself.

In the few times I was able to speak to Jenna the last few days, there are glimpses of light in what felt like the darkest darkness I will ever experience.

She would frequently inform the doctors that she was DNR (do not resuscitate), she would mention "how awful would it be to be with Jesus and then wake up back here in all this pain."

She had no fear.

She spoke of the great banquet she was going to attend and "*eat all the food*" and to run again. To the very end, she was not shy to share how excited she was to go and be with Jesus. In fact, just weeks prior, the only complaint I ever heard her say was when she was feeling terrible, "*This sucks, I want to go and be with Jesus.*"

Her heart was right where it needed to be. At peace and eagerly waiting to be with her Savior.

On Sunday October 2nd 2016, at 2:12 am, Jenna came face to face with the One whom she LOVED and gave herself to; and she was fully restored and fully healed.

No more pain, no more tears. The life Jesus promises us was fully revealed to her on that day.

Jesus says,

*"I am the resurrection and the life. Anyone who believes in me will live, even after dying. Everyone who lives in me and believes in me will never ever die. Do you believe this?"* [1]

### John 11:25, 26 (NLT)

In the past months, rarely does a minute go by where I am not grieving. Sorrow is found easy and often. It lurks at every turn. Questions and doubts come and go.

Yet I am surrounded by an amazing community of friends and family that are determined to walk, sit, and lament alongside me in this. Each day comes with different challenges, a journey which I may share in future blog posts, should I feel there is something of depth to share.

As I read through books Jenna found comforting, I stumbled across a highlighted passage in Tim Keller's book *Walking with God through Pain and Suffering*:

*"Now I have found freedom in anchoring my days and nights with Jesus' spirit. To live one day at a time without fretting over tomorrow frees me and soothes my suffering.*

*With renewed trust in Jesus comes renewed love, hope, and faith. My focus turns from my pain to His love. I have discovered a new treasure—the gift of pain is the gift of God Himself. In the end, He alone is truly my delight and comfort. I have learned the meaning of Psalm 119:71: "It was good for me to be afflicted so that I might learn your decrees."*

*Psalm 27:4 will now guide my journey till the end "One thing I ask of my Lord, this is what I seek: that I may dwell in the House of the Lord all the days of my life, to gaze upon the beauty of the Lord, and to seek Him in His temple."* [2]

I can say with confidence; this has been Jenna's heart through this journey. She suffered joyfully, something I hope to learn from her as a final gift she left for me to receive. Her confidence in Jesus speaks volumes and was displayed by the way she lived; by the way she suffered.

As I near the end of my writing, this was written to share the gap between Jenna's last post and October 2$^{nd}$. After that came another whirlwind of events and emotions in itself.

Thank you all for your continued prayers, the meals, the visits, the tears and the laughs, as I no doubt need them often.

Forever Grateful,
Scott

———

*"All their life in this world and all their adventures had only been the cover and the title page: now at last they were beginning Chapter One of the Great Story which no one on earth has read: which goes on forever: in which every chapter is better than the one before."* [3]

- C. S. Lewis

# Dear Mom,

Mom,

If you are reading this, that means your worst nightmare has come true. I want you to know that for me, this has been the thing I've been looking forward to with joy.

I know that is hard to believe, but when I started following Jesus in 2001, I became an heir to all the promises listed in the Bible. I mean all of them. There are some pretty awesome promises listed. Enough that if you read them all in one sitting, you'd be jealous of my situation right now.

I hope that someday you're able to see it like that, because that is one concrete thing in life. The only concrete thing. My God and the promises He has for his people ...

Love you, Jenna

# Epilogue

There was a deep, lasting ache that occurred when my wife, Jenna, passed away. A very real, very physical feeling of indescribable heaviness. I have no explanation for this other than a spiritual void left by losing a very piece of myself.

As time passes, so does the continuous weight felt in my chest. That's not to say it isn't there anymore, as it certainly is noticeable when I allow myself the quietness and the space. When I focus on myself, when I focus on what this life means to me now that this has all happened, it is easy for me to become overwhelmed with sorrow, depression, and apathy. Self-pity takes over and life becomes short-sighted; all about me, here and now.

But, when I focus on Jesus and His promises, suddenly the outlook changes. Sorrow turns to hope, depression turns to joy, and apathy turns to purpose. This temporary and unforgiving world is exchanged with an eternal world where things are set right forever. This is my hope, this is my joy. How can I not share this good news with everyone? How can I not center my life around the very One who promises us everlasting life? Jenna's death has, if anything, simplified and defined what matters most in this life—my relationship with Jesus.

This isn't to say every day is easy. It's not. It's quite the opposite. There are many days when all I want to do is embrace Jenna and share with her all that has happened since she left this world. I want to hear her voice tell me she loves me and that everything is going to be okay again, but I know those are deeply raw longings I will never get to experience again in this lifetime. Oh, how thankful I am that I am not left in this mess, and that Jesus promises He will, in His own timing, make all things new again.

Jenna's legacy goes well beyond the impact she had on my life and those who were close with her. She made it known that after her death, she wanted her tumor to be used to help those who would also face this awful disease. In honor of her wishes, her tumor was sent to Children's Minnesota, where a team of amazing people (who had also been working on treatments during Jenna's bout with cancer) continue to research and discover new ideas about how to tackle this cancer. Here is a glimpse of some of these developments:

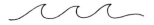

Dear Jenna,

I realize we've never met in person so what I'm about to write may seem a bit strange, but in truth you have inspired much of my current life's work. It is your story and that of a few others that make it clear how far we have yet to go in this work on dicer1 related tumors and especially dicer1 related ovarian tumors.

Specifically, you've taught us, taught me, about slct, neuroendocrine tumors and dicer1. From that one standpoint alone, I know you have saved lives. More people with neuroendocrine tumors will be screened now for dicer1 and if we find it, we stand a far better chance of detecting ppb in their relatives in its earliest and most crucial form. Those Jenna, are mostly kids under the age of 7, spared chemo and radiation, thanks to you.

Those are kids who, without you, would have had chemo, radiation, and still a survival rate of 53%, but instead will undergo surgery alone with a survival rate of 91%. Those babies, those children, are one of your many legacies. You've helped them the way you've helped so many others during your time here.

Even now, your tumor tissue is being used to test new therapies. At the moment, we're testing let-7 MiRNA mimics—we don't know if it will work yet. If it doesn't, and even if it does, our next step is to test locked nucleic acids— with the idea that someday those could be given to "lock-off" that DNA strand containing the "second hit."

You inspire all of this and you inspire all of us. I am so grateful for your work and your generosity during the most challenging journey life can offer. Despite your youth, your reach far exceeds what any of us has done in our lifetimes.

Thank you. With gratitude and prayers,

*- Kris Ann S.*

———

Since receiving this letter, I continue to receive periodic updates about their progress. It is truly humbling to know that the very thing Jenna so passionately wanted—to give kids a hope to defeat cancer—is one of the very things she is still doing.

Additionally, Jenna continues to also leave her legacy as a Young Life leader. A memorial endowment fund has been set up in Jenna's name to provide annual scholarships to kids who would otherwise not be able to attend camp. Ever since Jenna gave her life to Jesus at a Young Life camp, she has been passionate about sharing God's love with teenagers. She devoted her life to reaching kids with the Gospel and believed the best way to do that was to take kids to Young Life camp every year. Young Life camp gives kids the opportunity to hear about God in terms that they can understand, gives them the opportunity to spend time with their leaders, who care about and listen to them, and provides an opportunity for them to respond to Christ's love.

By purchasing this book, know that some of the proceeds are given towards these causes. If you feel led to donate directly to either of these missions, you can find out more at www.WorthTheSuffering.com. Also on this website, you will find many of the photos, videos, and links mentioned in this book.

I want to thank you all from the bottom of my heart for reading about Jenna's story. My hope is that no matter what you may be suffering through, you too can persevere through it with joy and hope, just as Jenna did, as she leaned heavily on Jesus.

# Afterword

I'm continually reminded of the day my brother Scott first told me about Jenna. We were walking on the beach as Scott described who would soon become the love of his life. Everything about her felt pure and perfect. I couldn't wait to meet her.

I sensed unease as Scott began to tell me more. As he shared the story of Jenna's prior battles with cancer, it became very real to me that he had already played some unwanted scenarios through his mind. God was already at work, nudging him, challenging him, and preparing him. Never did I expect that unspoken fear would be relived.

I can never be thankful enough for his brave pursuit of Jenna. She blessed our family in so many ways—which brings tears to my eyes as I reflect. I've realized that God's work through others happens in unimaginable ways. Jenna truly was a tangible example of what it looks like to follow Jesus.

It is because of her that my own purpose is stronger today and I am grateful for that. Jenna lived her life for Jesus and continues to inspire, encourage, and influence me to believe each and every day.

As you continue on this daily journey we call life, remember to do so with courage and hope. Live like Jenna, devote yourself to a greater purpose, and hold on to her words, "*I love that,*" no matter what situation you find yourself in.

*- Ryan H.*

# Acknowledgments

Family and friends, I am beyond grateful for you. Words feel shallow when I try to express the depth of my gratitude for you through this journey. From the moment we received news that Jenna's cancer had returned, you were there. You spent countless hours driving to be with us, you donated thousands of dollars to help cover our financial burdens, you prayed fervently when we asked (and even when we did not), you delivered hot meals without request. You were present.

When the weight of Jenna's death crushed me, you stepped into the deepest darkest pits with me—without hesitation. You sat with me, you cried with me, you doubted with me, and you spoke truth to me. Many of you delayed your own grieving to step in and carry burdens you didn't have to, keeping me from further despair. Even further, some of you put your own lives on hold just to be with me that first week.

As the months passed, and I felt the Lord calling me to share Jenna's story through a book, you gave me so much encouragement and excitement to move forward.

To all of you who shared a story about your friendship with Jenna, thank you. Thank you for allowing your heart to access that difficult place and share a glimpse of your relationship with Jenna. With your stories, this book represents a more complete picture of what life with authentic friendship looks like.

Ryan, thank you for slowing me down in this process, and for speaking up when God was giving you direction and vision for this book. Your words made this book what it is today and were exactly what I needed to hear at exactly the right time.

Leah, thank you for loving Jenna well as your sister. She cared deeply for you and connected with you in so many ways. I am honored and thankful for your work on the cover design and the insights you provided to make this book display Jenna's creativity in its design.

And finally, to my wife.

Jenna, you have done so much for my heart and my character. I am different now, a better man now, because of you. I am forever grateful for the moments we shared together, for the memories that I pray will never fade, and for the ways you *ALWAYS* pointed me back to Jesus. It hurts deeply to think about you not being here with me now, but your joy and hope in Jesus reminds me that this present life is temporary.

Your heart for everlasting life through Jesus is such a gift and such a blessing. It refocuses me every time I think about you. You were intentional with me even as you were physically struggling and mentally exhausted.

You said to me, *"Promise me you will never stop following Jesus,"* and though at the time I had a hard time responding confidently in the face of reality, it stays with me to this day and is a reminder I need often. Oh, how I cannot wait to see you again and share with you *"all the things."*

It feels tragic that it took this situation to finally understand the depth of the words *"I Love You."* The last words I spoke to you remain forever unchanged. I love you so so much.

Friends and family, thank you from the bottom of my heart.

With Love,
*Scott*

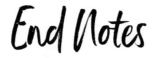

# End Notes

**Worth the Suffering**
Written by Jenna Henderson, *Jenna Nicole Photography*, www.jennanicolephotography.com.

**Foreword**
1.   "About Young Life," Young Life, accessed October 20, 2017, http://www.younglife.org/about.
2.   Galatians 5:22, 23 (NLT)

## ARRIVING STORMS

**Only the beginning**
1.   James 1:12 (NIV)
**Where it all started**
1.   Isaiah 42:16 (NIV)
**You've Never Failed**
1.   "Oceans" Copyright © 2013 Hillsong Music Publishing (APRA) (adm. the US and Canada at CapitolCMGPublishing.com) All rights reserved. Used by permission.
2.   Isaiah 43:2 (NIV)
3.   Matthew 14:25-33 (ESV)
**Treatment Plans**
1.   Lyrics from the song *You Are Mine* by Karla Adolphe, from the *Enter The Worship Circle* album: *Chair and Microphone, Vol. 3*, used by permission.
2.   Philippians 4:7 (ESV)
**Revelation Song**
1.   Kari Jobe, "Revelation Song."
**What a Week**
1.   Quote by Elisabeth Elliot.
2.   1 Samuel 12:16
3.   Acts 16:25 (ESV)
**First Chemo Down**
1.   Taken from *Every Bitter Thing is Sweet* by Sara Hagerty Copyright © 2014 by Sara Hagerty. Used by permission of Zondervan. www.zondervan.com.
2.   Matthew 16:24 (ESV)
3.   *Your Hands by JJ Heller, David Heller, and Katie Herzig.* From the album *Painted Red.* Used by permission.
**Hair Loss & Truth**
1.   Taken from *Every Bitter Thing is Sweet* by Sara Hagerty Copyright © 2014 by Sara Hagerty. Used by permission of Zondervan. www.zondervan.com.
**Roots to Grow Deep**
1.   John 11:4 (ESV)
**Present in the Sorrows**
1.   1 Samuel 12:16 (ESV)
**2nd Chemo Down & Young Life Camp**
1.   Taken from *Restless* by Jennie Allen Copyright © 2013 by Jennie Allen. Used by permission of Zondervan. www.zondervan.com.
**A Video for Your Sunday**
1.   Steven Manuel, *God is a Streetfighter*, Crossroads Church, https://www.crossroads.net/message/3581/A-Street-Fighter.
2.   Quote by Steven Manuel.
**Answered Prayers & Peaches**
1.   Daniel 3:17, 18 (NLT)

**Difficult Decisions**
1.     Hosea 6:3 (NLT)
**The Middle**
1.     Taken from *Bittersweet* by Shauna Niequist Copyright © 2010 by Shauna Niequist. Used by permission of Zondervan. www.zondervan.com.
2.     William Cowper, *God Moves in a Mysterious Way.*
**Make the Rough Places Smooth**
1.     Genesis 39:21-23 (ESV)
**Chemo #5 Down & Radiation Started**
1.     Ruth 4:14 (ESV)
**Final Stretch**
1.     Taken from *When God Doesn't Fix It* by Laura Story Copyright © 2015 by Laura Story. Used by permission of Zondervan. www.zondervan.com.
**After Chemo**
1.     *Harry Potter and the Prisoner of Azkaban*: Copyright © J. K. Rowling 1999. Used by permission.
**Chemo Is Finished!**
1.     Mark 4:39 (ESV)
**Not Quite Out of The Woods**
1.     Isaiah 40:2 (NIV)
2.     Isaiah 40:28-31 (NIV)
**My Last Radiation**
1.     Psalm 27:8 (NIV)


## EXHALE
**Finished**
1.     Taken from *Bittersweet* by Shauna Niequist Copyright © 2010 by Shauna Niequist. Used by permission of Zondervan. www.zondervan.com.
**Left with Scars**
1.     Housefires, "Good Good Father."
2.     Galatians 6:17 (NIV)
**Real Intimacy**
1.     Isaiah 6:8 (ESV)
**An Internal Struggle**
1.     Luke 1:45 (ESV)
**Fear Can't Win**
1.     Taken from *Every Bitter Thing is Sweet* by Sara Hagerty Copyright © 2014 by Sara Hagerty. Used by permission of Zondervan. www.zondervan.com.
**5 Months Out**
1.     Excerpt(s) from *Walking with God Through Pain and Suffering* by Timothy Keller, copyright © 2013 by Timothy Keller. Used by permission of Dutton, an imprint of Penguin Publishing Group, a division of Penguin Random House LLC. All rights reserved.
2.     Colossians 2:7 (NIV)


## CRASHING WAVES
**Cancer Is the Worst**
1.     Philippians 4:7 (NIV)
**The Rough Plan**
1.     John Piper, *Don't Waste Your Cancer* (Wheaton, IL: Crossway Books, 2011). Used by permission.
2.     Taken from *"The Happy Hour"* with Jamie Ivey. Happy Hour #68: Jami Nato [podcast]. Available at http://jamieivey.com/happy-hour-68-jami-nato. Used by permission.
**Prayers on Easter**
1.     John 11:25, 26 (NLT)
**Before Surgery**
1.     Zephaniah 3:17 (ESV)
**Post-Surgery Update**
1.     *The Voyage of the Dawn Treader* by CS Lewis © copyright CS Lewis Pte Ltd 1952. Used by permission.

271

**Raging Storm**
1.    Psalm 116:2 (NLT)

**Chemo Update + Turning 30**
Matthew 14:28, 29 (ESV)

**It's Different This Time**
1.    Margaret Feinberg, *Fight Back with Joy* Taken from *Fight Back with Joy* by Margaret Feinberg. Copyright © 2015 by Margaret Feinberg. Used by permission.

**Worst News**
1.    Psalm 107:29, 30 (NLT)
2.    Isaiah 38-40 (ESV)

**Fly Your Banner High**
1.    Isaiah 43:18-21 (ESV)
2.    Isaiah 43:19 (ESV)

**Peace in the Storm**
1.    Proverbs 30:5 (NIV)

**While on Vacation**
1.    Psalm 119:50 (ESV)
2.    Ephesians 6:15 (NIV)

**Life Since the Bad News**
1.    Daniel 3:17, 18 (NIV)
2.    Excerpt(s) from *Walking with God Through Pain and Suffering* by Timothy Keller, copyright © 2013 by Timothy Keller. Used by permission of Dutton, an imprint of Penguin Publishing Group, a division of Penguin Random House LLC. All rights reserved.
3.    Taken from *One Thousand Gifts* by Ann Voskamp Copyright © 2010 by Ann Morton Voskamp. Used by permission of Zondervan. www.zondervan.com.

**You More Than Anything**
2 Corinthians 4:16-18 (ESV)

**Half My Life**
1.    Isaiah 26:19 (NLT)

**Treatment & Life Update**
1.    Deuteronomy 31:8 (ESV)
2.    Video found at www.WorthTheSuffering.com.
3.    Rend Collective, "My Lighthouse."

**Glimpses of You**
1.    Matt Chandler, *The Result: Justification, Adoption and Sanctification*, http://www.tvcresources.net/resource-library/sermons/the-result-justification-adoption-and-sanctification. Used by permission.

**Shine Through**
1.    *A Long Obedience in the Same Direction* by Eugene H. Peterson. Used by permission.

**Everyone Must Know**
1.    2 Corinthians 4:12 (ESV)
2.    2 Corinthians 4:14 (ESV)

**Focus My Heart**
1.    2 Corinthians 3:2, 3 (ESV)
2.    Philippians 1:21 (ESV)
3.    1 Corinthians 15:55 (NIV)

**Long Update & Young Life Camp**
1.    Psalm 119:50 (ESV)
2.    Taken from *Restless* by Jennie Allen Copyright © 2013 by Jennie Allen. Used by permission of Zondervan. www.zondervan.com.
3.    Quote by Justin Ryder, "Young Life Staff and podcast." Used by permission.

**Scans and The Plan**
1.    2 Corinthians 1:9, 10 (ESV)
2.    Psalm 51:7, 8 (ESV)

**One Last Entry**
1.    Psalm 27:4 (NLT)

**The Last Battle**
1.    *The Last Battle* by CS Lewis © copyright CS Lewis Pte Ltd 1956. Used by permission.
2.    John 11:25, 26 (NLT)
3.    Excerpt(s) from *Walking with God Through Pain and Suffering* by Timothy Keller, copyright © 2013 by Timothy Keller. Used by permission of Dutton, an imprint of Penguin Publishing Group, a division of Penguin Random House LLC. All rights reserved.